the COMPLETE GUIDE to FASTING

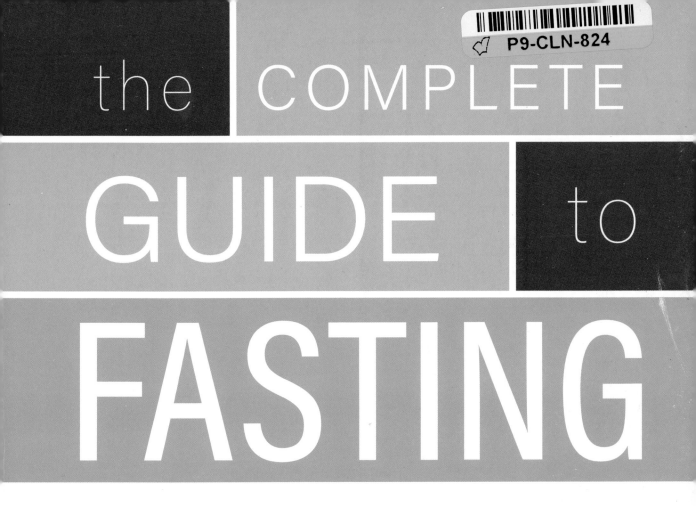

Heal Your Body Through *Intermittent, Alternate-Day,* and *Extended* Fasting

Jason Fung, MD · *with* Jimmy Moore

Victory Belt Publishing
Las Vegas

First Published in 2016 by Victory Belt Publishing Inc.

ISBN 13: 978-1-628600-01-8

Book design by Justin-Aaron Velasco
Illustrations by Justin-Aaron Velasco
Food photography (recipes) by Tom Estrera
Food preparation and styling by Luzviminda Estrera

Printed in Canada
TC1118

CONTENTS

INTRODUCTION
by Jason Fung, MD

I grew up in Toronto, Canada, and studied biochemistry at the University of Toronto, where I also completed medical school and my residency in internal medicine.

After my residency, I chose to study nephrology (kidney disease) at the University of California, Los Angeles, mostly at Cedars-Sinai Medical Center and West Los Angeles VA Medical Centers (then known as the VA Wadsworth). Each field of internal medicine draws its own personalities, and nephrology has the reputation of being a "thinker's specialty." Kidney disease involves intricate fluid and electrolyte problems, and I enjoy these puzzles. In 2001 I returned to Toronto to start my career as a nephrologist.

Type 2 diabetes is far and away the leading cause of kidney disease, and I treat many hundreds of patients with this disease. Most type 2 diabetics also suffer from obesity. By the early 2010s my interest in puzzles, combined with my professional focus on obesity and type 2 diabetes, had led me to focus on diet and nutrition.

How did I go from preaching conventional medicine to prescribing intensive dietary strategies, including fasting? Despite what you might think, nutrition is not a topic covered extensively in medical school. Most schools, including the University of Toronto, spend a bare minimum of time teaching nutrition. There were perhaps a handful of lectures on nutrition in my first year of medical school and virtually no teaching on nutrition throughout the rest of medical school, internship, residency, and fellowship.

Out of the nine years spent in formal medical education, I would estimate I had four hours of lectures on nutrition.

As a result, I had no more than a passing interest in nutrition until the mid-2000s. At the time, the Atkins diet, promoting low-carb eating, was in full swing. It was everywhere. Some family members of mine tried it and were ecstatic with the results. However, like most conventionally trained physicians, I believed their arteries would eventually pay the price. I, along with thousands of other physicians, had been taught and certainly believed that low-carbohydrate diets were simply a fad and the low-fat diet would prove to be the best.

Then studies on the low-carb diet started to appear in the most prestigious medical journal in the world, the *New England Journal of Medicine*. Randomized controlled trials compared the Atkins diet to the standard low-fat diet that most health-care providers recommended. These studies all came to the same startling conclusion: the low-carb diet was significantly better for weight loss than the low-fat diet. Even more stunning was that all the important risk factors for cardiovascular disease—including cholesterol, blood sugar level, and blood pressure— were also much improved on the low-carb diet. This was a puzzle, a real conundrum. And that was where my journey began.

Figuring Out What Causes Obesity

The new studies proved that the low-carb approach was a viable one. But this didn't make any sense to me because I was still steeped in the conventional "calories in, calories out" (CICO) approach—the idea that the only way to lose weight is to consume fewer calories than you expend. Diets based on the Atkins methodology, for example, did not necessarily restrict caloric intake, yet people were still losing weight. Something didn't add up.

One possibility was that the new studies were wrong. However, that was unlikely, given that multiple studies all showed the same result. Furthermore, they confirmed the clinical experience of thousands of patients, who were all reporting weight loss on the Atkins diet.

Logically, accepting that the studies were correct meant the CICO approach had to be wrong. Much as I tried to deny it, there was no saving the CICO hypothesis. It was dead wrong. And if the CICO hypothesis was wrong, then what was right? What caused weight gain? What was the etiology—the underlying cause—of obesity?

Doctors spend almost no time thinking about this question. Why? Because we think we already know the answer. We think that excessive caloric intake causes obesity. And if eating too many calories is the problem, then the solution is eating fewer calories and burning more through an increase in activity. This is the "eat less, move more" approach. But there's an obvious problem. "Eat less, move more" has been done to death over the past fifty years, and it doesn't work. For all practical purposes, it doesn't really matter *why* it doesn't work (although we'll look into that in Chapter 5); the bottom line is that we've all done it, and *it doesn't work*.

The underlying cause of obesity turns out to be a *hormonal*, rather than a caloric, imbalance. Insulin is a fat-storage hormone. When we eat, insulin increases, signaling our body to store some of this food energy as fat for later use. It's a natural and essential process that has helped humans survive famine for thousands of years, but excessively and persistently high insulin levels result inexorably in obesity. Understanding this leads naturally to a solution: if excessive insulin is causing obesity, then clearly the answer lies in reducing insulin. Both the ketogenic diet (a low-carb, moderate-protein, high-fat diet) and intermittent fasting are excellent methods of reducing high insulin levels.

Insulin and Type 2 Diabetes

However, in my work with type 2 diabetics, I realized that there was an inconsistency between the treatment of obesity and the treatment of type 2 diabetes, two problems that are closely linked. Reducing insulin may be effective in reducing obesity, but doctors like me were prescribing insulin as a cure-all treatment for diabetes, both types 1 and 2. Insulin certainly lowers blood sugars. But just as surely, it causes weight gain. I finally realized that the answer was really quite simple. We were treating the wrong thing.

Type 1 diabetes is an entirely different problem than type 2. In type 1 diabetes, the body's own immune system destroys the insulin-producing cells in the pancreas. The resulting low insulin level leads to high blood sugar. Therefore, since insulin levels are low to begin with, it makes sense to treat the problem with supplemental insulin. And sure enough, it works.

In type 2 diabetes, however, insulin levels are not low but *high*. Blood sugar is elevated not because the body can't make insulin but because it's become resistant to insulin—it doesn't let insulin do its job. By prescribing more insulin to treat type 2 diabetes, we were not treating the underlying cause of high blood sugar: insulin resistance. That's why, over time, patients saw their type 2 diabetes get worse and required higher and higher doses of medications.

But what caused the high insulin resistance in the first place? This was the real question. After all, we didn't stand a chance of treating the underlying disease if we didn't know what caused it. As it turns out, *insulin causes insulin resistance.* The body responds to excessively high levels of any substance by developing resistance to it. If you drink excessive alcohol, your body will develop resistance, up to a point—we often call this "tolerance." If you take narcotics such as heroin, your body will develop resistance. If you use prescription sleep medications such as benzodiazepines, your body will develop resistance. The same holds true for insulin.

Excessive insulin causes obesity, and excessive insulin causes insulin resistance, which is the disease known as type 2 diabetes.

With that understanding, the problem with how doctors treat type 2 diabetes became clear: we were prescribing insulin to treat it, when excessive insulin was the problem in the first place. Instinctively, most patients knew what we were doing was wrong. They would say to me, "Doctor, you have always told me that weight loss is critical in the treatment of type 2 diabetes, yet you have prescribed me insulin, which has made me gain so much weight. How is that good for me?" I never had a good answer for this. Now I knew why. They were absolutely right; it *wasn't* good for them. As patients took insulin, they gained weight, and when they did, their type 2 diabetes got worse, demanding more insulin. And the cycle repeated: they took more insulin, they gained more weight, and as they gained more weight, they needed more insulin. It was a classic vicious cycle.

We doctors had been treating type 2 diabetes *exactly* wrong. With the proper treatment, it is a curable disease. Type 2 diabetes, like obesity, is a disease of too much insulin. The treatment is to *lower insulin*, not raise it. We were making things worse. We were fighting the fire with gasoline.

I needed to help my obesity and type 2 diabetes patients lower their insulin levels, but what was the best approach? Certainly, there are no medications that do this. There are surgical options that help, such as bariatric surgery (commonly called "stomach stapling"), but they are highly invasive and have many irreversible side effects. The only feasible treatment left was dietary: reducing insulin levels by changing eating habits.

In 2012, I established the Intensive Dietary Management Program, which has a unique focus on diet as a treatment for the twin problems of obesity and type 2 diabetes. At first, I prescribed low and very low carbohydrate diets. Since refined carbohydrates highly stimulate insulin, reducing these carbohydrates should be an effective method of lowering insulin.

I gave my patients lengthy sessions of dietary advice. I reviewed their food diaries. I begged. I pleaded. I cajoled. But the diets just didn't work. The advice seemed hard to follow; my patients had busy lives and changing their dietary habits was difficult, especially since much of it ran contrary to the standard advice to eat low-fat and low-calorie.

But I couldn't just give up on them. Their health, and indeed their very lives, depended upon reducing their insulin levels. If they had trouble avoiding certain foods, then why not make it as simple as possible? *They could simply eat nothing at all.* The solution was, in a word, *fasting*.

NOT JUST ANOTHER F-WORD: MY EXPERIMENTS WITH FASTING
by Jimmy Moore

In the coming pages, you will read all about the therapeutic uses of fasting and how to implement it in your own life in order to experience its amazing health benefits. But you might be wondering what the experience of fasting actually looks like—perhaps particularly for someone who was extremely skeptical about fasting until he tried it for himself. That's precisely what I'll be sharing with you in this chapter. My name is Jimmy Moore, and I'm the internationally bestselling author of *The Ketogenic Cookbook*, *Keto Clarity*, and *Cholesterol Clarity*, as well as the host of the longest-running health podcast, *The Livin' La Vida Low-Carb Show with Jimmy Moore*. When I discovered Dr. Jason Fung's incredible work on fasting, I knew we needed to collaborate to get comprehensive information about fasting into the hands of as many people as possible. But I wasn't always such an exuberant fan of fasting.

"This Has Got to Be a Joke, Right?"

When I first heard about fasting as part of improving your overall health over a decade ago, it might as well have been described as "the other f-word." *Why in the world would you purposely starve yourself? How could anyone possibly think that deliberately being hungry would ever be a good thing? This has got to be a joke, right?* Believe me, I know many of you reading this book have had some of these exact same thoughts. And back in 2006, I didn't fully comprehend the positive benefits fasting would someday provide me, including its amazing effects on my cholesterol and blood sugar.

I first heard about the concept of intermittent fasting from Dr. Michael Eades, author of the bestselling book *Protein Power*. In 2006, Dr. Eades began writing about the great success with weight loss and other health benefits he had seen with something called intermittent fasting, or IF. It was a new idea at the time to go periods of time without eating anything at all, on a regular basis, and the way he described it seemed relatively doable: stop eating at 6:00 p.m. and then don't eat again until 6:00 p.m. the next day. So you still got to eat every single day, but this strategy forced your body to go without food for twenty-four hours at a time.

I have to admit, I had never gone that long without eating in my entire life, and I was extremely skeptical about the whole idea of fasting, even on an intermittent basis. Why? Because I like to eat, as evidenced by the fact that I once weighed in at a whopping 410 pounds. Of course, at that weight I was consuming lots of processed junk food and sugary sodas like there was no tomorrow. Growing up, in college, when I got married in my twenties, and into my early thirties, I had terrible eating habits that contributed to some pretty significant metabolic damage. Thankfully in 2004 I came across information about the low-carb diet, which enabled me to lose 180 pounds in one year and come off of three prescription medications for high cholesterol, high blood pressure, and breathing problems. I had to share the incredible health success I'd found on that diet with others, and I went on to grow a huge platform online called *Livin' La Vida Low-Carb*, which I use to educate, encourage, and inspire others in their own personal health journeys. I write books, give talks around the world, and speak with some of the most influential and intelligent people making waves in nutrition, fitness, and health. It's been some of the most gratifying work of my entire life, and I'm privileged to be able to do what I do for a living now.

Despite my diet turnaround, though, I didn't stop enjoying eating! Hence my skepticism about intermittent fasting. I was intrigued by what Dr. Eades had to say about it, though, and I did my homework. One thing I learned in particular made me sit up and take notice. In 2009, I interviewed Boston College biology professor Thomas L. Seyfried, who had been researching alternative treatments for cancer prevention and treatment, including using a calorie-restricted ketogenic diet to treat brain cancer and other cancers. One of the more interesting and memorable nuggets from that half-hour interview came at the very end of our conversation, when Dr. Seyfried made the bold assertion that an annual seven- to ten-day water fast could be a useful tool for preventing cancer. WOW! But as skeptical as I was about intermittent fasting, a one-week fast freaked me out even more. Who could actually do that?

But by that point I'd heard enough to convince me to give fasting a try. Needless to say, I had to get my head around IF before I even dared try a multiple-day fast, and being the nothing's-too-hard adventurer that I was, I decided to try it. Boy oh boy, what was I getting myself into?!

My First Attempt at Fasting

Okay, before we get to the good stuff about fasting, I have to be honest about the bad stuff, and all I have to say about my first attempt at alternate-day intermittent fasting—fasting for twenty-four hours every other day—is ugh, ugh, and UGH! It lasted exactly four days, nineteen hours, and fifteen minutes. *But it felt like an eternity!* I did some things wrong that made this attempt much more painful than it should have been, but before I explain what so that you can learn from my mistakes, here's what I learned about myself during my first, unpleasant experience of attempting IF in 2006:

1. I was pretty addicted to caffeine still. That first day of fasting was painful because I had a massive headache for most of the day. By the second day, though, the headache had subsided.

2. I hadn't felt truly hungry in a long time. After losing 180 pounds, my philosophy had been to never allow myself to get hungry so I didn't slip back into those old eating habits. (Ironically, during my low-fat dieting days, all I did was have hunger pangs.) Now, listening to my body is beneficial because I don't have the same food temptations.

3. Being ravenously hungry made me overeat. At the end of my second fasting day, my wife Christine and I went to Steak & Ale for their all-you-can-eat prime rib special. They were busy, so the steaks took longer to come to the table than they usually do. I was so hungry that I ate a whole plate of salad in minutes, devoured the first prime rib, waited twenty minutes for my second, and killed that one, too. Then my server brought me another one about thirty minutes later (after my food had settled a bit in my stomach) and I started to eat it—but when I got halfway done, *whoa Nelly*, I was full! Not just full, but *really really full!* As in, it hurt so much I had to take some Tum-ta-Tum-Tums and lie down for a bit when we got home. I was quite the ravenous beast!

4. Eating enough food to fuel my daily workouts really was important. On day 1 of my fast, I tried to keep up the same resistance and speed on my elliptical workout, but it just didn't happen. While I usually have a 13 resistance at 8.5 mph, I had to back off to 7 resistance at 7.0 mph to keep my workout as long as usual. Of course, I burned fewer calories as well. What was worse was that even on the days I *did* eat, the very noticeable lack of energy persisted, and my energy did not return until I ended my IF experiment. It took me several weeks to get back to full strength and endurance.

5. For me at the time, going without food for twenty-four hours was not realistic. On the first day my head was hurting so much from the caffeine withdrawals that I barely noticed how hungry and light-headed I felt. But on my second fasting day, I felt like I was floating around my office ready to tip over at any moment. My body was lethargic and I felt dissociated from everything, as if I wasn't in the living world. My coworkers kept asking me if I was okay because I wasn't my normal chipper self.

Call me a wimp for not making it through even one whole week on the IF experiment, but it was just not for me. And there are a few reasons why.

First, I was still drinking diet sodas during the fast, and that stoked hunger and cravings that I wouldn't have had otherwise. Second, I wasn't getting enough salt during the fast, which led to fatigue and energy drain. Better than those diet sodas would have been bone broth with sea salt, which provides much-needed electrolytes and is satiating. And finally, I just didn't have the right mindset. I didn't anticipate just how tough it would be at the beginning, and I wasn't prepared to handle the hunger—both real and imagined.

After this attempt at IF crashed and burned in a blaze of glory, I didn't think I'd try it again. But then in 2011, after some gentle prodding from people like Robb Wolf and other IF advocates, I decided to give it another go.

Success on IF, and a Growing Ambition

During this second attempt, I gave myself eighteen to twenty hours between meals, and it was much better for me than going twenty-four hours between meals. In fact, it was quite easy eating a meal in the morning around 9:00 a.m. and then another around 2:00 p.m. as the totality of my food intake for the day—so I fasted between 2 p.m. one day and 9:00 a.m. the next day, about nineteen hours. I even sometimes mixed it up and pushed my first meal to around 12:00 p.m. and then the second meal to 5:30 p.m. for a shorter feeding window. I felt very comfortable doing this and it became very natural to me.

I hadn't forgotten about the idea of an extended period of fasting as a way to boost my health, though. When I interviewed Dr. Thomas Seyfried on my podcast in 2009, he was adamant that a one-week fast would be beneficial as an annual cancer-prevention strategy. Of course, most people can't (or, more realistically, won't) do something like this. But what would it be like to actually try it for myself? Once IF started to come more naturally to me, in 2011, I decided it might be time to push the total fasting time to an entire week. Would I make it through a longer fast? I didn't know at the time, but today I'm so glad I put aside my fears and gave it the old college try.

In addition to my growing ease with IF, two things gave me the confidence to try an extended fast. First, one of my blog readers, who had done three one-week fasts over the span of a year on the suggestion of his doctor to help with some prostate issues, shared something with me that put things into perspective. Here's what he said:

> The way you experience yourself physically when you are fasting is practically identical to the way you experience yourself physically when you are eating. The reason this is so important is that when you think you experience hunger while eating normally, that same experience of hunger is present when you are fasting. In other words, the hunger sensations in fasting are the same as while eating normally. You then have to ask yourself how you can be hungry when you have eaten three hours ago when it is the same hunger sensation when you have not eaten anything at all for a week. What we think is hunger is not really hunger. That impulse to eat cannot be taken seriously.

Wow! So if we can learn to view hunger in the right way, then we can be more resistant to the temptations that inevitably befall so many of us during fasting. As my reader so succinctly put it, "fasting allows you to reclaim your hunger for what it is [so] it no longer dictates what you put in your mouth." Now that's a message I think we can all learn something from. By the way, the series of one-week fasts my reader completed was "tremendously successful" in treating those prostate issues he had. This helped convince me that fasting really is a powerful therapy.

The second thing that propelled me to do a one-week fast was that I'd been learning a lot about all the benefits of being in a state of nutritional ketosis—and fasting and ketosis go together perfectly, like bacon and eggs. When you eat a low-carb, moderate-protein, high-fat diet—a ketogenic diet—it becomes much easier to fast. The carbohydrate restriction and protein moderation help to keep your blood sugar and insulin levels under control, and consuming adequate amounts of healthy saturated and monounsaturated fats keeps your hunger at bay. And here's the key to why keto is so great for fasting: being in ketosis teaches your body to burn fat for fuel rather than sugar, and since that's what your body has to do during fasting, if you're already in ketosis, your body is already using fuel the way it's supposed to.

Think of it this way: You have at least 40,000 calories' worth of fat on your body right now, but only 2,000 calories' worth of sugar.

If you're a fat-burner, when you start fasting, your body simply continues to use fat as its primary fuel. If you're a sugar-burner, though, your body burns those 2,000 calories of sugar until it's all gone, and then it triggers hunger until it's adapted to using fat. As a sugar-burner, you'll feel the effects of hunger during a fast much earlier and more intensely. This is why going keto (covered in detail in my book *Keto Clarity*) is a great first step for fasting, both IF and extended fasting.

I wasn't quite in ketosis yet myself when I tried the one-week fast, but I had been eating low-carb for a long time, and I was reassured that my body could handle an extended fast.

Extended Fasting Take 1: A Week Without Food

On the evening of April 10, 2011, I consciously chose to do one of the most unlikely things I'd ever done in nearly four decades of living: I embarked on a one-week fast—*on purpose*—just to see how I would do.

So many people asked at the time if I was doing it to lose weight, and the answer was, *not at all*. Any weight loss on a complete extended fast (unlike on a regular IF routine) would not likely stay completely off once food was reintroduced. That's not to say a few stubborn pounds of fat wouldn't find a way to leave my body, and that's never a bad thing. But my primary purpose was to monitor how I felt going without any food for a week.

I learned so much more than I could have ever imagined.

The physical experience of the fast

The first three days were some of the most difficult because my body was screaming at me to eat something. I felt spacey for much of the time, as if everything around me was running in slow motion. But at the same time, my thoughts were clear and I was fully functioning, despite having had no food. And honestly, I felt good for most of the time throughout the entire fast. Days 4 and 5 were the best of the seven as I experienced the big whoosh of renewed energy that I had heard so many people share would happen. On day 6, though, I struggled early on with a strong desire to eat again, and by day 7, when I was at church and took communion, I felt absolutely horrible, like my blood sugar had dropped to a level that zapped me of all my energy. When I checked my blood sugar level and saw a reading in the 50s and could barely stand up around 2:00 p.m. on the final day of the fast, I knew it was time to break it.

Effects on blood sugar and weight

I didn't measure my blood sugar every single day, but the few times I did I saw readings in the 60s. Sure, this was below 80, the level I generally saw on my healthy low-carb lifestyle, but that's what happens when you don't eat any food at all. Controlling blood sugar and giving your pancreas a week to rest from producing insulin is an excellent reason for attempting a fast like this.

The first few days I lost about a pound a day, and then on days 4 to 7 I lost several pounds. While I wasn't doing this to lose weight, it certainly produced a sizable drop on the scale: thirteen pounds in one week. I learned later that the weight loss on a one-week fast like this is mostly water weight because the fasting process depletes glycogen stores.

Exercising

Believe it or not, I decided to keep up with my exercise routine during my fasting week, and I did a whole lot better than I thought. I knew not to push it too hard, and I told my wife that if I started to feel dizzy or anything, I would stop. Even still, I played competitive volleyball twice and did a couple of Pilates/yoga classes with no problems. Although I was spacey on the volleyball court, I was able to perform quite well, running, jumping, and blocking spikes in the front row!

The bathroom

Yes, I know it's gross to talk about, but it's a part of the fasting experience. I expected to visit the porcelain goddess frequently in the first couple of days or so, but when I was still seeing massive amounts of "stuff" coming out late in the week, that was pretty freaky—after all, I hadn't consumed anything in many days, so what was coming out? It reminded me that there's a lot more waste in the body than we even realize, and doing this fast may have helped clean a good bit of that out.

Nutritional supplements

I did not stop taking my regular supplements for the duration of the fast. I continued with my multivitamin, vitamin D3, magnesium, probiotics, and other vitamins that have been a part of my healthy low-carb lifestyle for years. Perhaps I could have given this routine a rest for a week, too, but I didn't.

How I made it through

This was my first attempt at fasting for longer than a day, so I didn't have any idea what to expect beyond what I had heard from others. One of the challenges I faced was how to ward off the symptoms of not eating anything—the light-headedness and lethargy I'd experienced on my first fast. I was guzzling a lot of water (very important for anyone who's fasting), but I decided I wanted more. So I added in some diet sodas to help get me through. While I no longer drink diet sodas, they were somewhat helpful in getting through the fast. (Yes, I know, Dr. Fung advises against this—see page 171—and they're probably a big reason why my first attempt at fasting was so tough. It's a journey we all need to take.) I also included bouillon cubes to help with electrolyte imbalance. I've since learned that a better, healthier way to get these helpful effects is to drink kombucha and bone broth with sea salt.

Other people's reactions

When I started sharing my fasting experience on social media, the reaction I received was probably the most surprising part of the entire fast. It ran all across the spectrum, from encouraging words from people who thought this was a great idea and cheered me on all the way to people telling me I was killing myself and undermining the very low-carb-lifestyle principles I promote. Some of the response was as if I'd used the other f-word in church!

What would I have done differently?

I hate to say I'd change anything about my first experience trying a one-week fast. The experience was what it was, and it was eye-opening. At the time, I planned to eat some coconut oil if the hunger became too much to bear, but it never did, and now I can't help but wonder if the addition of coconut oil or other strategies might have made a difference in the way I felt. Adding in these things might have stoked some hunger, but maybe not. It got me thinking about how to tweak and improve my fasting attempts in the future.

After the fast ended, I decided to write to the man who inspired this one-week fast—Dr. Seyfried himself—whom I had met in person that year at an obesity conference in Baltimore, Maryland. When I told him what I had done, he said he was happy to hear I "survived" my fasting experience. He said the vitamins I took and other things I added to my fast may have sent "mixed signals to the body," making the fast more difficult. Dr. Seyfried noted that a cancer-preventing fast should probably be done using distilled water only and nothing else. He also lamented that I didn't measure the level of ketones—byproducts of the body burning fat—in my blood. (I would learn more about that and start testing them one year later.) He suspected that my blood ketones were elevated, which helped me endure the fast for the week.

Dr. Seyfried was so impressed by my experiment that he included it in his textbook on cancer, *Cancer as a Metabolic Disease: On the Origin, Management, and Prevention of Cancer*. Here's what he wrote:

> Mr. Jimmy Moore also described his experience with a seven-day, mostly water-only fast in a podcast video. Mr. Moore is a well-known blogger for the health benefits of low-carbohydrate diets. He was able to document the physiological changes he experienced during the fast in nontechnical language. Although Mr. Moore followed most of what Herbert Shelton would consider standard practices, Mr. Moore included bouillon cubes in the fast. Chicken and beef bouillon contain some calories and salts, which might prevent glucose from reaching the lowest levels needed to put maximum metabolic pressure on tumor cells. However, Mr. Moore's blood

glucose levels did fall within the required therapeutic ranges for tumor management during his fast. Further research is needed to document the influence of bouillon and other low-calorie and low-carbohydrate food items on blood glucose and ketone levels during food fasting. Nevertheless, it is important for cancer patients to recognize from Mr. Moore's podcast that fasting is not harmful.

Combining Fasting and Nutritional Ketosis

Fast-forward to 2012, when I began my one-year experiment with nutritional ketosis. By eating a low-carb, moderate-protein, high-fat diet, I was able to switch my body from primarily burning glucose for fuel to burning fat. As part of the experiment, I started keeping track of my blood ketones, as Dr. Seyfried had suggested.

I had no intention at all of fasting as part of the ketosis experiment. But I quickly discovered that it just started happening spontaneously and naturally, especially when my blood ketone levels exceeded 1.0 millimole. I remember that early on, in the first few weeks of my experiment, my wife asked me when the last time I ate was. After looking at the clock and then going back through my food logs, I discovered it had been about twenty-eight hours. I had totally forgotten to eat. In light of my history of eating, this was absolutely stunning!

Once my body made the switch from burning glucose to burning fat, the idea of eating breakfast, snack, lunch, snack, dinner, snack, midnight snack just seemed silly. Why would I want to eat that often when I wasn't hungry? My body was very clearly telling me it was okay that I didn't think about food that obsessively anymore. We simply aren't meant to be eating as much or as often as we

AMY BERGER ▮ FASTING ALL-STARS

I prefer for my clients to stick to a good, nutrient-dense low-carb diet and get fat-adapted for a while before experimenting with fasting. I think it's easier and more pleasant to fast when your body isn't still screaming out for carbohydrates.

do in modern culture, and getting into ketosis by consuming real, whole foods on a diet that is low-carb, moderate-protein, and high-fat, with adequate calories, will allow you to spontaneously fast for twelve to twenty-four hours. (Read my book *Keto Clarity* to learn more about how going ketogenic can make intermittent fasting a cinch.)

My main point here is that when I got into a state of nutritional ketosis—when I became mostly a fat-burner rather than a sugar-burner—fasting became completely natural for me. Of course, many of you reading this aren't eating a ketogenic diet or pursuing nutritional ketosis, and that's fine (although you should be!). Dr. Fung has had a lot of success using fasting as a therapeutic approach with many of his patients who aren't in ketosis. But my own experience with fasting has been that it was difficult before I got into ketosis, and perfectly natural and easy afterward.

That one-week fast really showed me the power of the ketones in keeping me completely energized and comfortable during a fast. Even though I wasn't in ketosis when I started the fast, *during* the fast my body was burning fat and producing ketones, and it felt great. That's the bottom line to remember—once you're accustomed to fasting, it happens very naturally and shouldn't be associated with much hunger or discomfort after the first few times. And the advice in this book will help you get through those first few times, which I admit can be tough. But tough doesn't mean impossible. My first fasting experience was terrible, but now I can do it on a whim, and it feels great. The only thing I can tell you to do is try it yourself and watch what happens. It's incredibly freeing to not think about food twenty-four hours a day, seven days a week, 365 days a year. Is it still sounding like another f-word to you now?

What happens if you do get hungry or don't feel good while intermittent fasting? Ummmm, hello, McFly? You *eat* something! This isn't rocket science, people. While it's normal to have some hunger and discomfort for the first couple of days, there's a difference between minor discomfort and the I'm-going-to-literally-bite-someone's-head-off-if-I-don't-eat-something discomfort. If your energy is just gone and not coming back, or you're not feeling like yourself, or you're insanely hungry, don't push through. Fasting shouldn't be physically painful. End it, have something to eat, and try again in a week or so.

Of course, as my blog reader shared, true hunger is much different than what we have come to expect. The sad fact is, most people don't listen to what their body is telling them. Instead, they eat more out of habit, comfort, and boredom than anything else. This is critical to understand if you're going to attempt to engage in fasting.

If you've never done IF before, then a twenty-four-hour period with no food can sound absolutely torturous. Your body is used to getting food at certain times of the day and will send not-so-subtle cues that it is time to eat. I used to think that was true hunger, but it's really not. Instead, it is simply your body's internal clock trying to keep you on your normal, familiar routine of eating. But does that mean we are supposed to succumb to the desire to eat when that feeling hits? I used to think so, but the wisdom of experience has now taught me the answer is an emphatic *no*. The fact is that our stomach can remain quite satisfied even when everyone else around us is chowing down on food because it's "time to eat."

When I weighed over 400 pounds, prior to 2004, I felt like I was hungry virtually all the time, no matter how much food I put in my mouth. Getting my hunger under control and recognizing what true hunger feels like was a huge part of my eventual success and still sustains me all these years later.

There are plenty of people like me who can comfortably eat one or two meals a day without a problem thanks to nutritional ketosis, so we can go through periods of fasting quite naturally. But I will tell you now that there will be social challenges associated with fasting. If your friends or family want to gather together for a meal and you're either not hungry or engaged in an extended fast, then some people just don't know how to handle it. You don't want to be rude at the gathering, and the host doesn't want to feel they did something wrong. Remember, these occasions aren't really about the food as much as they are about connecting with others. Focus on the connections and let them stuff their face with whatever they want. Most people will hardly notice you aren't eating. And if they do, it's their problem, not yours. Of course, the best thing to do is to plan your fast around celebrations and events where food is important. Don't start a seven-day fast three days before a birthday party or wedding. But for everyday, spur-of-the-moment get-togethers, try to behave normally and enjoy the company without fixating on the food.

Extended Fasting Take 2: A Three-Week Fast

After my success formally testing the ketogenic diet in 2012 and 2013, which led to a deeper understanding of nutritional ketosis, I thought it would be useful to try fasting again. Of course, I didn't need to "try" IF—I was doing it practically on a daily basis because ketosis made it so easy—so I decided to revisit longer fasting to see if I could go beyond a week. I met Dr. Jason Fung in February 2015, and after learning about the work he was doing with over a thousand patients, using various fasting protocols to improve their health, I was intrigued by the idea of fasting for more than one week. Could I make it for twenty-one days in a row this time around?

In September 2015, I set out on a twenty-one-day fast with only water, kombucha, and bone broth with sea salt, together totaling well under 200 calories daily. While technically this was not a pure fast, since there was some minimal caloric intake, Dr. Fung advised me that I would get most of the benefits of a water-only fast with this protocol. I shared daily updates during the fast on my Periscope channel. Predictably, my weight came down very quickly, as did my blood sugar levels—they went into the 70s and even upper 60s with no signs of hypoglycemia. I checked my blood ketones as well, and while they started at very low levels, they catapulted to well above 2.5 millimoles by day 4 of the fast. I felt euphoric and surprisingly energetic—unlike the previous time I did a longer fast!

My first day of fasting was extremely easy because I was already used to fasting for twenty-four hours with my ketogenic diet. Day 2 was the most difficult for me—the desire to eat was much more intense than I had expected. But then something incredible happened once I got past the second day: fasting became surprisingly simple! It was almost *too* easy to just not eat.

The notion that if you don't eat, you'll experience an increasing feeling of hunger the longer it lasts, is simply not true. In fact, I daresay that after fasting for a few days, you will actually feel more *normal* than perhaps you ever have before. And when you don't think so much about what you'll eat, when you'll eat, where you'll eat, and all the other social customs surrounding food, it frees you up to do other things. You'll realize the urge and desire to eat is more mental than physical.

So how did my twenty-one-day fasting attempt go? I made it a total of seventeen and a half days, only to be sabotaged by something that I really didn't expect: stress from traveling. My wife and I went on vacation with friends in Myrtle Beach, South Carolina, beginning on day 15 of the experiment, and by the evening of day 17, my stomach was growling for forty-five minutes straight! Because it was close to bedtime, I decided to wait until the next morning to see if the hunger would dissipate. It did not, and so I broke the fast just a few days short of my original goal. But I listened to my body, and that is always very important when you are fasting.

It's not a big deal to end the fast when it becomes obvious the time to stop fasting has come. I'd fasted for nearly three times longer than I ever had in my life, so I was pretty stoked. But the fact that I had to stop showed me just how profoundly impactful stress can be, and now I've started taking active measures to reduce stress in my life—meditation, less time online, yoga classes, and regular massages all help. Because I have severe insulin resistance due to years of poor nutrition, I think stress probably impacts me more than most. If I can figure out this piece of the health puzzle, then maybe a book called *Stress Clarity* could be in my future. Stay tuned!

ROBB WOLF ▪ FASTING ALL-STARS

Fasting *is* a stress. Whether it is a hormetic (beneficial) stress or potentially a detrimental stress is largely determined by what other life stressors are at play.

Predictably, I lost weight on this fast: nineteen pounds. While that wasn't its primary purpose, it was a nice little side effect. Most fascinating to me was the fact that sixteen pounds had stayed off when I checked one month after I ended the fast. That was pretty cool. And because I'm such a nerd when it comes to health markers, I of course ran a series of blood tests before and after my seventeen-and-a-half-day fast to see what impact the fasting had. Some of these results were predictable, but others took me totally by surprise. Here's what happened to various blood markers prior to and immediately after my fast:

	PRE-FAST	POST-FAST
Total cholesterol	295	195
LDL-C	216	131
HDL-C	61	50
Triglycerides	90	68
LDL-P	2889	1664
Small LDL-P	1446	587
Lp(a)	441	143
Fasting insulin	13.9	10.0
hsCRP	1.6	.94

Most of those numbers are related to cardiovascular health, including advanced cholesterol tests. (You can learn more about cholesterol numbers in my 2013 book *Cholesterol Clarity*.) But let me interpret what happened here. Did you see anything that kind of stuck out more than others? Yep, it was the cholesterol. Total cholesterol dropped 100 points in less than three weeks of fasting, without the need for any cholesterol-lowering medications like statin drugs. As patients, we're often told that drugs are the only way to get our cholesterol down so we won't have a heart attack, and yet here is a totally drug-free method for lowering cholesterol.

My HDL-C, known as the "good" cholesterol, predictably fell from 61 to 50 during the fast. One of the basic materials needed for HDL cholesterol is fat, especially saturated fat. So when you don't consume any food at all, you can expect your HDL to drop. But most of the reduction in the total cholesterol number was in the LDL-C, which dipped from 216 to 131, but this doesn't tell the entire story about the improvements to my heart health. Fasting did something I've never seen any pharmaceutical drug do before.

The advanced lipid panel known as an NMR lipoprofile test shows the actual number of LDL particles and the size of those particles. When I began my fast, the total LDL particles (LDL-P) was 2889 and the small LDL-P (the truly bad LDL) was 1446. After the fast, these numbers dropped to 1664 and 587, respectively, representing a significant improvement. But perhaps the most stunning result of all of these tests was the Lp(a) (Lipoprotein a), a risk factor in the development of cardiovascular disease. My initial Lp(a) of 441 was extremely high (always has been), and it plummeted to 143. That's a powerful indication of the therapeutic effects of fasting.

The final two blood tests were for fasting insulin and hsCRP (high-sensitivity C-reactive protein), a key inflammation marker. The good news is that these numbers weren't bad before I started and only got better after the fast. There was a nearly four-point drop in the fasting insulin, and my hsCRP fell almost in half.

All in all, the numbers showed that my three-week fast was a great success. But I wasn't finished yet.

Extended Fasting Takes 3, 4, and 5: Another Week, Fasting Cycles, and a Month Without Food

In mid-October 2015, I did another fast for one week to see if I would see similar changes in my key markers. Interestingly my blood sugar fell once again into the 70s and 80s, and I lost 13.4 pounds. However, that weight didn't stay off this time around. Perhaps I am one of those people who need longer fasts to see the results stick.

My next fasting experiment took place in December 2015, when I tried cycling the fasting with some nonfasting days to see how that would work for me. I fasted for six days, then ate on day 7, fasted another five days, then ate on day 13, then fasted another four days, and ended the fast. It was fun changing things up a bit, but I didn't see the same results doing this as I did with the nearly three-week consecutive fast. My blood sugar and blood ketone levels never improved to the levels I'd come to expect from an extended fast. That said, I lost 18.2 pounds and had kept off five pounds of it when I checked a month later. But I had one more idea for a fast that would be my most controversial one of all.

In January 2016, I had the idea to fast for the entire month. Yep, you heard me right. I wanted to fast for thirty-one days in a row. It was daunting, but I'd been encouraged by the results of my two previous extended fasts, so I decided to give it a go. This time around, I thought it would be fun to have a dual-energy X-ray absorptiometry scan—better known as a DXA scan—run to see what happened to my body fat and muscle mass during this fast. Several of my followers on social media were concerned that I was losing massive amounts of muscle on these fasting experiments. So I was scanned before and after the January 2016 fast. More on those results in a moment.

I was going along swimmingly on this fast, seeing fabulous improvements in my blood sugar, which plummeted down into the 70s and 60s again, and blood ketones, which were well over 2.5 millimolar again, and I was feeling fantastic. In fact, on day 11 I decided to test my blood sugar and blood ketones every hour on the hour to see what was going on. The results are in the table on page 28.

Those are some pretty spectacular numbers, and I was feeling incredible throughout the day, despite having not eaten for eleven days in a row at that point.

On day 13, I needed to pause the fast and eat because we were driving to Virginia to be with my wife's family. Once again, the stress bug bit me hard, and it took a toll on my ability to fast. Thankfully I got right back on it after taking one day off and was doing well until three days later, when we needed to drive home. Once again, the stress caused me to pause the fast for a second time. During travel, hunger, weakness, and a general feeling of blah just hit me like a ton of bricks, and I know not to ignore that feeling. So I again ate on day 16 and began the fast again the next day. I fasted for six more days after that, paused one last time on day 22, and then made it the final nine days of the month. All in all, I fasted twenty-eight of the thirty-one days in January 2016.

Although my blood sugar and blood ketone levels were up and down because I had to pause the fast occasionally, I still lost 22.4 pounds and kept off fourteen of it in the month that followed.

Time	Blood glucose	Blood ketones	Food consumed
7:30 a.m.	66	3.1	
8:30 a.m.	67	3.1	-
8:45 a.m.	-	-	Kombucha
9:30 a.m.	72	3.9	-
10:30 a.m.	70	2.9	-
10:30 a.m.	-	-	Chicken bone broth with sea salt
11:30 a.m.	73	2.9	-
12:30 p.m.	71	2.6	-
1:30 p.m.	70	3.8	-
2:30 p.m.	68	4.3	-
3:30 p.m.	79	3.8	-
4:30 p.m.	71	3.7	-
5:30 p.m.	72	4.2	-
6:30 p.m.	68	3.9	-
7:30 p.m.	60	4.7	-
8:30 p.m.	62	4.5	-
9:30 p.m.	74	3.7	-

And what about those DXA scan results? Now this was fascinating. The scan showed I lost ten pounds of body fat and another ten pounds of what it identified as "lean tissue," generally interpreted as muscle. All of this supposed "muscle loss" happened in the trunk area; I actually gained muscle in my arms and legs. When I discussed this result with Dr. Fung, he noted that the DXA scan can mistake fat loss in organ tissues for muscle loss. In other words, most likely I lost not muscle but rather fat around my internal organs—a very good thing!

So I returned to my low-carb, ketogenic way of eating for a couple of weeks and had the DXA scan run again. What happened to that lean tissue it showed I lost during my fast? Every single pound of that so-called muscle loss was completely gone and I was back to the level I was at prior to the fast. It just goes to show you that these measurements are merely tools and should never lead to false assumptions. The fact is, I didn't lose any muscle during my twenty-eight days of fasting, and that's pretty remarkable! It goes against everything commonly believed about the side effects of fasting. (Dr. Fung discusses the myth that fasting causes muscle loss in more detail on page 75.)

Conclusion: A Fasting Fan!

I'm still tweaking my own personal fasting protocol, taking into account that I probably need longer fasts to receive the most benefits and that, as I've learned, it is incredibly important for me to try not to fast during stressful times, even when it's happy stress. Traveling makes longer-term fasting a no-go for me (although I will easily do an intermittent fast if the flight is under four hours), and so do any out-of-the-ordinary activities, such as writing books or attending conferences. This is a great lesson I learned from my fasting escapades.

If you're now inspired to give fasting a try for yourself, let me encourage you to just do it. Even if you begin by simply skipping lunch, you can work your way up to fasting for a few days in a row, and the benefits will be tremendous. Dr. Fung will talk in more detail about those benefits in the coming chapters, but suffice to say, if you're struggling with obesity and/or type 2 diabetes, fasting can have an incredible effect on weight and blood sugar. I've seen it with my own eyes, even when I was still skeptical about fasting.

I understand that it can be a real challenge to not eat for a period of time. It's especially tough because in our modern world, food is instantly available on every street corner. But what if you decided to buck the trend, abstain from eating even for a short period of time, and see how you do? Forget about what you think *might* happen and instead embrace the experience to see what *does* happen. I'm not going to tell you it will solve all of your weight and health issues. It's certainly not a cure-all. But fasting can become one of the most practical tools that can empower you to take back control of your own health. That's a goal we should all be striving for!

Meet the
FASTING ALL-STARS

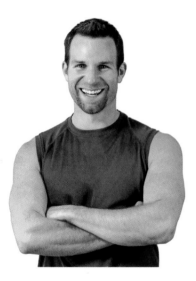

Abel James is a *New York Times* bestselling author and modern-day Renaissance man. He stars as a celebrity coach on ABC Television and has been featured in *People* magazine, *WIRED*, *Entertainment Tonight,* and *NPR.* As host of the number-one podcast in more than eight countries, *Fat-Burning Man,* Abel has helped millions reclaim their health and perform at their best with cutting-edge science, outdoor workouts, and outrageously good food.

Abel has keynoted for the federal government, lectured at Ivy League universities, and advised Fortune 500 companies, including Microsoft, Danaher, and Lockheed Martin. He was named one of the 100 Most Influential People in Health and Fitness by Greatist in 2015 and 2016.

Distinguished as a Senior Fellow with Honors at Dartmouth College, Abel created his own curriculum to specialize in brain science, music, and technology. He later published his research in *The Musical Brain,* which became a number-one bestseller.

Also a songwriter and multi-instrumentalist, Abel has won several awards in writing and performance arts, including "Outstanding Achievement in Songwriting."

Abel lives with his wife in Austin, Texas. He enjoys strong coffee and cheesecake, preferably together. Visit his website, fatburningman.com, for more.

Amy Berger, MS, CNS, NTP, is the author of the book *The Alzheimer's Antidote*. She has a master's degree in human nutrition and is a Certified Nutrition Specialist and Nutritional Therapy Practitioner. As a US Air Force veteran, she has a special interest in the use of low-carbohydrate and ketogenic diets for neurological health (including traumatic brain injury), as well as improving metabolic conditions such as type 2 diabetes and obesity.

After spending years doing what health and nutrition experts claimed were "all the right things" to lose weight and maintain optimal health and failing to experience the expected results, Amy discovered that the conventional advice about low-calorie, low-fat dieting and exercise did not lead to the promised outcomes. In pursuing training in nutrition and physiology, she learned that much of what we currently believe about "healthy diets" is misguided and, in many cases, downright incorrect.

Having learned these lessons the hard way, Amy has dedicated her career to showing others that vibrant health does not require starvation, deprivation, or living at the gym. Men and women cannot live by lettuce alone. *Real people need real food!* You can read her blog and find more of her work at tuitnutrition.com.

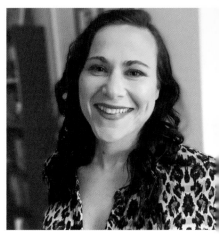

Dr. Michael Ruscio helps people identify why they are sick and helps them get well naturally. He works with patients across the country, utilizing lab-based natural medicine treatments to help a variety of patients, from athletes to the chronically ill, overcome health problems and achieve optimal health and well-being. Visit his website, DrRuscio.com, for more.

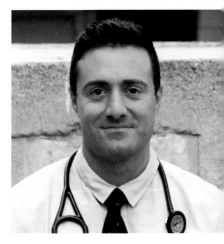

DR. BERT HERRING

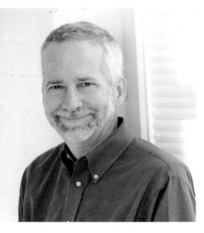

Bert Herring, MD, ("Dr. Bert") pioneered daily intermittent fasting, first experimenting with it himself in 1995, then studying it further and sharing it with the world in 2005 with the first guide to starting and reaping the benefits of a daily fasting/eating cycle, *The Fast-5 Diet and the Fast-5 Lifestyle*.

Dr. Bert's focus is on real-world solutions: things that work for real people with real lives and real commitments, like kids and jobs. He pays attention to what works for people who can't exercise eight hours per day, and he keeps his skepticism high when it comes to results that only concern lab rats, short-duration studies of only a few weeks' duration, and studies in which people are being observed (because, as Heisenberg said, observation changes things).

Dr. Bert also has little interest in temporary solutions. Temporary solutions may work, but if you can't sustain them, they can't become part of your lifestyle. He wants to arm people with the tools necessary to fight culture's drives to overeat and help them build a customized, low-hassle way of living that achieves a healthy balance and works for the long term.

Health goes far beyond diet, so Dr. Bert does too. To see more, look for his TEDx talk, "Did I Enrich Today?," which has over 235,000 views, or visit his website, bertherring.com.

MEGAN RAMOS

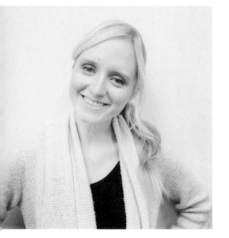

Megan Ramos worked with Dr. Fung for over sixteen years as a medical researcher prior to cofounding the Intensive Dietary Management Program. Having helped hundreds of patients incorporate fasting into their lives, there is likely nobody else in the world with her clinical expertise. Visit intensivedietarymanagement.com for more.

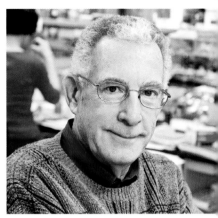

Thomas N. Seyfried is a professor of biology at Boston College and received his PhD in genetics and biochemistry from the University of Illinois, Urbana, in 1976. He did his undergraduate work at the University of New England, where he recently received the distinguished Alumni Achievement Award. He also holds a master's degree in genetics from Illinois State University. He was a postdoctoral fellow in neurology at the Yale University School of Medicine and then served on the faculty as an assistant professor in neurology. Thomas Seyfried served with distinction in the US Army's First Cavalry Division during the Vietnam War and received numerous medals and commendations.

Other awards and honors have come from such diverse organizations as the American Oil Chemists Society, the National Institutes of Health, the American Society for Neurochemistry, and the Ketogenic Diet Special Interest Group of the American Epilepsy Society. Dr. Seyfried previously served as chair of the Scientific Advisory Committee for the National Tay-Sachs and Allied Diseases Association and presently serves on several editorial boards, including those for *Nutrition & Metabolism*, *Neurochemical Research*, *Journal of Lipid Research*, and *ASN Neuro*, where he is a senior editor. Dr. Seyfried has over 170 peer-reviewed publications and is the author of *Cancer as a Metabolic Disease: On the Origin, Management, and Prevention of Cancer*. His full list of peer-reviewed publications can be found on PubMed (ncbi.nlm.nih.gov/pubmed).

MARK SISSON

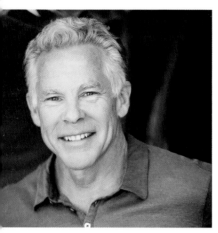

Mark Sisson is the author of the bestselling book *The Primal Blueprint*, as well as *The Primal Blueprint Cookbook* and the top-rated health and fitness blog *MarksDailyApple.com*. He is also the founder of Primal Kitchen, a company devoted to designing, manufacturing, and distributing healthy, great-tasting food products made with clean proteins, healthy fats, and no sugars.

ROBB WOLF

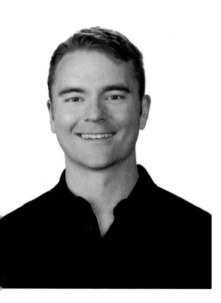

Robb Wolf, a former research biochemist, is the *New York Times* bestselling author of *The Paleo Solution: The Original Human Diet*. A student of Professor Loren Cordain, author of *The Paleo Diet*, Robb has transformed the lives of hundreds of thousands of people around the world via his top-ranked iTunes podcast, book, and seminars.

Robb has been a review editor for the *Journal of Nutrition and Metabolism*, is cofounder of the nutrition and athletic training journal *The Performance Menu*, is co-owner of NorCal Strength & Conditioning, one of the *Men's Health* top 30 gyms in America, and is a consultant for the Naval Special Warfare Resiliency program. He serves on the board of directors/advisors for: Specialty Health Inc., Paleo FX, and *Paleo Magazine*.

Robb is a former California State Powerlifting Champion (565 lb. squat, 345 lb. bench, 565 lb. dead lift) and a 6–0 amateur kickboxer. He coaches athletes at the highest levels of competition and consults with Olympians and world champions in MMA, motocross, rowing, and triathlon. Robb has provided seminars in nutrition and strength and conditioning to a number of entities, including NASA, Naval Special Warfare, the Canadian Light Infantry, and the United States Marine Corps.

Robb lives in Reno, Nevada, with his wife, Nicki, and daughters Zoe and Sagan. Visit his website, robbwolf.com, to learn more.

FEARS

—forget them

ADVANTAGES

—so many

SCHEDULE

—whenever you need it

THERAPEUTIC

—for so many health concerns, like obesity, diabetes, cancer, and Alzheimer's

Part One

WHAT IS FASTING
AND WHY IS IT GOOD FOR YOU?

Chapter 1
WHAT IS FASTING?

Mentioning fasting as a treatment for obesity and type 2 diabetes always gets the same eye-rolling response. *Starvation? That's the answer? You're going to starve people?* No. That is not it at all. I'm not going to starve people; I'm asking them to fast.

Fasting is completely different from starvation in one crucial way: control. Starvation is the *involuntary* abstention from eating. It is neither deliberate nor controlled. Starving people have no idea when and where their next meal will come from. This happens in times of war and famine, when food is scarce. Fasting, on the other hand, is the *voluntary* abstention from eating for spiritual, health, or other reasons. Food is readily available, but you *choose* not to eat it. No matter what your reason for abstaining, the fact that fasting is voluntary is a critical distinction.

Starving and fasting should never be confused with each other, and the terms should never be used interchangeably. Fasting and starving live on opposite sides of the world. It is the difference between recreational running and running because a lion is chasing you. Starvation is forced upon you by outside forces. Fasting, on the other hand, may be done for any period of time, from a few hours to months on end. You may begin a fast at any time of your choosing, and you may end a fast at will, too. You can start or stop a fast for any reason, or for no reason at all.

Fasting has no standard duration—since it is merely the absence of eating, anytime that you are not eating, you are technically fasting. For example, you may fast between dinner and breakfast the next day, a period of twelve hours or so. In that sense, fasting should be considered a part of everyday life. Consider the term *breakfast*. The word refers to the meal that "breaks your fast"—which is done daily. The word itself implicitly acknowledges that fasting, far from being some sort of cruel and unusual punishment, is performed daily, even if only for a short duration. It is not something strange but a part of everyday life.

I've sometimes called fasting the "ancient secret" of weight loss. Why? It is certainly an ancient technique, dating thousands of years, as we'll discuss in Chapter 2. Fasting is as old as humankind, far older than any other dietary technique. But how is fasting a "secret"?

Although fasting has been practiced for millennia, it has been largely forgotten as a dietary therapy. There are virtually no books about it. There are few websites dedicated to fasting. There is almost no mention of it in newspapers or magazines. Even its very mention draws stares of incredulity. It is a secret hiding in plain sight. How did this happen?

Through the power of advertising, big food companies have slowly changed how we think of fasting. Instead of being a purifying, healthful tradition, it's now seen as something to be feared and avoided at all costs. Fasting was extremely bad for business, after all—selling food is difficult if people won't eat. Slowly but inevitably, fasting has become forbidden. Nutritional authorities now allege that even skipping one single meal will have dire health consequences.

You must always eat breakfast.

You must snack constantly, all day long.

You should eat a bedtime snack.

You must never, ever miss a meal.

These messages are everywhere—on television, in the newspaper, in books. Hearing them over and over again creates the illusion that they are absolutely true and scientifically proven beyond a doubt. The truth is exactly the opposite. There is no correlation whatsoever between constant eating and good health.

Sometimes authorities will try to convince you that you can't fast because you'll be consumed by hunger. It's too difficult. It is simply impossible. Here, the truth is also the exact opposite.

I had certainly read a ton on the anti-aging benefits of fasting, but I was hesitant to try it for myself, fearing I might lose precious muscle mass. Then, on a long overseas flight, with no food available and not having eaten since the previous night, I was forced into a 36-hour fast. I found myself completely energetic and clear-headed. Based on that experience, I started experimenting with how long I could go without eating (actually, without feeling like I *had* to eat). I found it could be quite long periods of time. I also noticed that I didn't lose mass or strength, which was key for me.

Can you fast? Yes—it's been done by literally millions of people around the world, for thousands of years.

Is it unhealthy? No. In fact, it has *enormous* health benefits.

Will you lose weight? If you don't eat anything for a day, do you think you will lose weight? *Of course.*

Fasting is effective, simple, flexible, practical, and virtually guaranteed to work. Ask a child how to lose weight, and she will probably say to skip a few meals. So what's the problem? Nobody makes money when you fast. Not Big Food. Not Big Pharma. Nobody wants you to find out the ancient secret of weight loss.

The Disappearance of Daily Fasting

In the 1970s, a typical American ate three meals a day—breakfast, lunch, and dinner, with no snacks. Data compiled from the National Health and Nutrition Examination Survey (NHANES) showed an average of three eating opportunities per day. I grew up in the 1970s and remember it well. What would happen if we tried to get an after-school snack? Usually there would be a slap on the hand and an admonition that "you'll ruin your dinner."

A typical day might include breakfast at 8:00 a.m., lunch at noon, and dinner at 6:00 p.m. That means that we would be eating for ten hours of the day, which is nicely balanced by fourteen hours of fasting. And guess what? Obesity and type 2 diabetes were not nearly the problems they are today.

Figure 1.1. The average number of meals and snacks consumed by adults increased from 3 per day in 1977–78 to almost 6 per day in 2003–06.

1977–1978 ━━━━
1994–1996 ━━━━
2003–2006 ━━━━

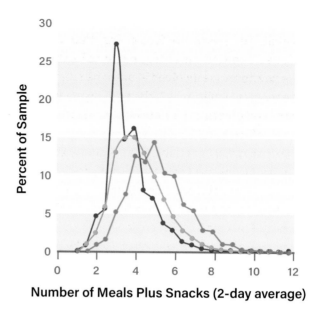

Source: Popkin and Duffey, "Does Hunger and Satiety Drive Eating Anymore?"

Fast-forward to today. Instead of trying to stop snacking, we actively *encourage* it in both adults and children. Some even feel that snacking more will help lose weight, as ridiculous as that sounds. Consider my son's typical schedule. He eats breakfast the moment he wakes up. There's a mid-morning snack at school, then lunch, then an after-school snack, dinner, and then another snack between halves of his soccer game, and then maybe a bedtime snack. He's eating six or seven times a day! This is by no means atypical. The NHANES data shows that the average American eats five or six times per day.

So instead of having balanced periods of feeding and fasting, we are now eating perhaps sixteen to eighteen hours of the day and only fasting for six to eight hours. Is it any wonder that obesity has become an epidemic?

To examine the reasons that fasting is more beneficial than most people think, let's start by looking at what actually goes on in the body when we eat and when we fast.

What Happens When We Eat?

When we eat, we ingest more food energy than we can immediately use. Some of this energy needs to be stored away for later. The key hormone involved in both the storage and use of food energy is insulin, which rises during meals. Both carbohydrates and protein stimulate insulin. Fat triggers a far smaller insulin effect, but it's rarely eaten alone.

Insulin has two major functions. First, it allows the body to immediately start using food energy. Carbohydrates are absorbed and rapidly turned into glucose, raising blood sugar levels. Insulin allows glucose to enter directly into most cells of the body, which use it for energy. Proteins are broken down into amino acids and absorbed, and excess amino acids may also be turned into glucose. Protein does not raise blood glucose, but it can raise insulin levels. The effect is variable, and it surprises many people to learn that some proteins can stimulate insulin as much as some carbohydrate-containing foods. Fats are directly absorbed as fat and have minimal effect on insulin.

Second, insulin helps store the excess energy. There are two ways to store the energy. Glucose molecules can be linked into long chains called glycogen and then stored in the liver. There is, however, a limit to the amount of glycogen that can be stored away. Once this limit is reached, the body starts to turn glucose into fat. This process is called *de novo lipogenesis* (literally, "making fat from new").

This newly created fat can be stored in the liver or in fat deposits in the body. While turning glucose into fat is a more complicated process than storing it as glycogen, there is no limit to the amount of fat that can be created.

EAT FOOD > increase INSULIN > STORE SUGAR IN LIVER / PRODUCE FAT IN LIVER

| NO FOOD "FASTING" | > | decrease INSULIN | > | BURN STORED SUGAR |
| | | | | BURN BODY FAT |

What Happens When We Fast?

The process of using and storing food energy that occurs when we eat goes in reverse when we fast. Insulin levels drop, signaling the body to start burning stored energy. Glycogen (the glucose that's stored in the liver) is the most easily accessible energy source, and the liver stores enough to provide energy for twenty-four hours or so. After that, the body starts to break down stored body fat for energy.

So you see, the body really only exists in two states—the fed (high-insulin) state and the fasted (low-insulin) state. Either we are storing food energy or we are burning food energy. If eating and fasting are balanced, then there is no net weight gain.

If, however, we spend the majority of the day storing food energy (because we're in the fed state), then over time, we will gain weight. What is needed then is to restore balance by increasing the amount of time we burn food energy (by going into the fasted state).

The transition from the fed state to the fasted state occurs in several stages, as classically described by George Cahill, one of the leading experts in fasting physiology:

1. *Feeding:* Blood sugar levels rise as we absorb the incoming food, and insulin levels rise in response to move glucose into cells, which use it for energy. Excess glucose is stored as glycogen in the liver or converted to fat.

2. *The postabsorptive phase* (six to twenty-four hours after beginning fasting): At this point, blood sugar and insulin levels begin to fall. To supply energy, the liver starts to break down glycogen, releasing glucose. Glycogen stores last for approximately twenty-four to thirty-six hours.

3. *Gluconeogenesis* (twenty-four hours to two days after beginning fasting): At this point, glycogen stores have run out. The liver manufactures new glucose from amino acids in a process called *gluconeogenesis* (literally, "making new glucose"). In nondiabetic persons, glucose levels fall but stay within the normal range.

4. *Ketosis* (two to three days after beginning fasting): Low insulin levels stimulate lipolysis, the breakdown of fat for energy. Triglycerides, the form of fat used for storage, are broken into the glycerol backbone and three fatty acid chains. The glycerol is used for gluconeogenesis, so the amino acids formerly used can be reserved for protein synthesis. The fatty acids are used directly for energy by most tissues of the body, though not the brain. The body uses fatty acids to produce ketone bodies, which are capable of crossing the blood-brain barrier and are used by the brain for energy. After four days of fasting, approximately 75 percent of the energy used by the brain is provided by ketones. The two major types of ketones produced are beta-hydroxybutyrate and acetoacetate, which can increase over seventyfold during fasting.

5. *The protein conservation phase* (five days after beginning fasting): High levels of growth hormone maintain muscle mass and lean tissues. The energy for basic metabolism is almost entirely supplied by fatty acids and ketones. Blood glucose is maintained by gluconeogenesis using glycerol. Increased norepinephrine (adrenaline) levels prevent any decrease in metabolic rate. There is a normal amount of protein turnover, but it is not being used for energy.

In essence, what we are describing here is the process of switching from burning glucose to burning fat. Fat is simply the body's stored food energy. In times of low food availability, stored food is naturally released to fill the void. The body does not "burn muscle" in an effort to feed itself until all the fat stores are used up. (More on this myth in Chapter 3.)

One critical point to underscore is that these mechanisms are entirely natural and entirely normal. Periods of low food availability have always been a natural part of human history, and our body evolved mechanisms to adapt to this fact of Paleolithic life. Otherwise, we would not have survived as a species. There are no adverse health consequences to activating these protocols,

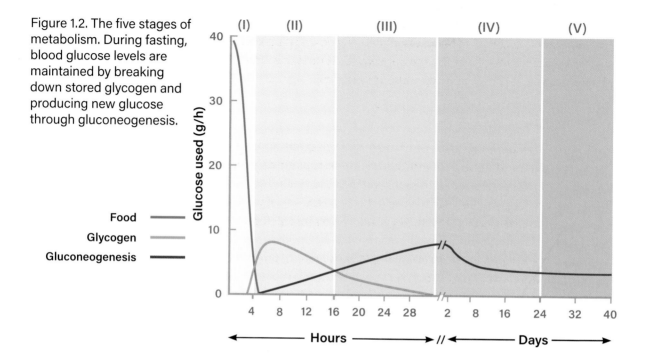

Figure 1.2. The five stages of metabolism. During fasting, blood glucose levels are maintained by breaking down stored glycogen and producing new glucose through gluconeogenesis.

	Feeding (I)	Postabsorptive Phase (II)	Gluconeogenesis (III)	Ketosis (IV)	Protein Conservation (V)
Origin of Blood Glucose	Food	Glycogen Gluconeogenesis	Gluconeogenesis Glycogen	Gluconeogenesis	Gluconeogenesis
Tissues Using Glucose	All	All except liver. Muscle and adipose tissue at diminished rates.	All except liver. Muscle and adipose tissue at rates intermediate between II and IV.	Brain, red blood cells, renal medulla. Small amount by muscle.	Brain at a diminished rate, red blood cells, renal medulla
Major Fuel of Brain	Glucose	Glucose	Glucose	Glucose, ketone bodies	Ketone bodies, glucose

Source: Cahill, "Fuel Metabolism in Starvation."

except in the case of malnourishment (you should not fast if you're malnourished, of course, and extreme fasting can cause malnourishment, too). The body is not "shutting down"; it's merely changing fuel sources, from food to our own fat. It does this with the help of several hormonal adaptations to fasting.

Insulin Goes Down

A decreased insulin level is one of the most consistent hormonal effects of fasting. All foods raise insulin to some degree. Refined carbohydrates tend to raise insulin the most and fatty foods the least, but insulin still goes up in both cases. Therefore, the most effective method of reducing insulin is to avoid all foods altogether.

During the initial stages of fasting, insulin and blood glucose levels fall but remain in the normal range, maintained by the breakdown of glycogen as well as gluconeogenesis. After glycogen is used up, the body begins to switch over to burning fat for energy. Longer-duration fasts reduce insulin more dramatically.

Regularly lowering insulin levels leads to improved insulin sensitivity—your body becomes more responsive to insulin. The opposite of insulin sensitivity, high insulin resistance, is the root problem in type 2 diabetes and has also been linked to a number of diseases, including:

Heart disease

Stroke

Alzheimer's disease

High cholesterol

High blood pressure

Abdominal obesity

Nonalcoholic steatohepatitis (fatty liver disease)

Polycystic ovary syndrome

Gout

Atherosclerosis

Gastroesophageal reflux disease

Obstructive sleep apnea

Cancer

Figure 1.3. Extended fasting over 4 days leads to decreased insulin and blood sugar levels.

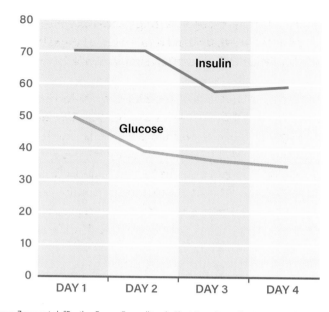

Source: Zauner et al., "Resting Energy Expenditure in Short-Term Starvation Is Increased as a Result of an Increase in Serum Norepinephrine."

Lowering insulin also rids the body of excess salt and water because insulin is well known to cause salt and water retention in the kidneys. This is why low-carbohydrate diets often cause diuresis, the loss of excess water—in fact, much of the initial weight lost on a low-carb diet is water. This diuresis is beneficial in reducing bloating and helping you feel lighter. Some may also note a lower blood pressure.

Electrolytes Remain Stable

Electrolytes are certain minerals in the blood. They include sodium, chloride, potassium, calcium, magnesium, and phosphorus. The body keeps these blood levels under very tight control in order to maintain health. Prolonged studies of fasting have found no evidence of electrolyte imbalances—the body has mechanisms in place to keep electrolytes stable during fasting.

Sodium and chloride: These minerals are found primarily in salt. Daily salt requirements are quite low, and most of us exceed this by many orders of magnitude. During short-term fasts, salt depletion is not a concern. During prolonged fasting (more than one week), the kidneys are able to reabsorb and retain most of the salt needed by the body. However, rarely, some salt supplementation may be required.

Potassium, calcium, magnesium, and phosphorus: Potassium levels may decrease slightly during fasting, but they'll remain in the normal range. Magnesium, calcium, and phosphorus levels are also stable during fasting. The bones carry large stores of these minerals—99 percent of what's in the human body. Normally some minerals are lost in the stool and urine, but during fasting, that loss is minimized. However, in children and pregnant and breastfeeding women there is an ongoing demand for these minerals, so fasting is not advisable.

Other vitamins and minerals: The daily use of a general multivitamin supplement will provide the recommended daily amount of micronutrients. A therapeutic fast of 382 days was maintained with only a multivitamin with no harmful effects on health. In fact, this man felt terrific during this entire period.

In a study of supervised fasts with only water and vitamins lasting up to 117 days, researchers confirmed that there were no changes in serum electrolytes, lipids, proteins, or amino acids. Moreover, they found that hunger was virtually absent during these prolonged fasts.

Adrenaline Increases and Metabolism Speeds Up

Most people expect that a period of fasting will leave them feeling tired and drained of energy. However, the vast majority of people experience the exact opposite: they feel energized and revitalized during fasting.

Partly this is because the body is still being fueled—it's just getting energy from burning fat rather than burning food. But it's also because adrenaline is used to release stored glycogen and to facilitate fat-burning, even if blood sugar is high. The increased adrenaline levels invigorate us and stimulate the metabolism. In fact, studies show that after a four-day fast, resting energy expenditure increased by 12 percent. Rather than slowing the metabolism, fasting revs it up.

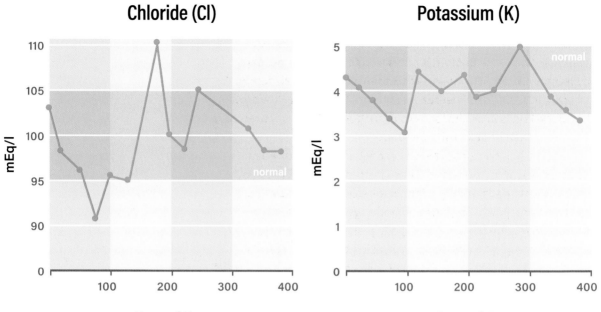

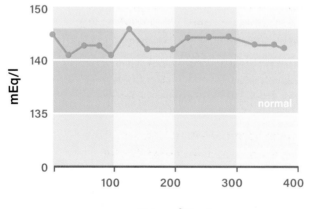

Figure 1.4. Electrolytes remain
stable during extended
fasting.

Source: Data from Stewart and Fleming, "Features of a Successful Therapeutic Fast of 382 Days' Duration."

Growth Hormone Goes Up

Human growth hormone (HGH) is made by the pituitary gland. As the name implies, it plays a huge role in the normal development of children and adolescents. Levels peak during puberty and gradually decrease with age. Excessively low growth hormone levels in adults leads to more body fat, less muscle mass, and decreased bone density (osteopenia).

Growth hormone, along with cortisol and adrenaline, is a counterregulatory hormone. These hormones signal the body to increase the availability of glucose—countering the effect of insulin and producing higher blood sugar levels. Levels of counterregulatory hormones peak just before waking, at approximately 4:00 a.m. or so, increasing blood sugar levels, which fall during the night. The increase prepares the body for the upcoming day by making more glucose available for energy.

Growth hormone also increases the availability of fats for fuel by raising levels of key enzymes, such as lipoprotein lipase and hepatic lipase. Since burning fat reduces the need for glucose, this helps maintain stable blood sugar.

Many of the effects of aging may result from low growth hormone levels. Replacing growth hormone in older people with low levels has significant anti-aging benefits. A randomized controlled study found that in men, six months of growth hormone replacement increased lean mass (bone and muscle) by an astounding 3.7 kilograms (8.2 pounds), even as fat mass *decreased* by 2.4 kilograms (5.3 pounds). Similar results were found in women.

However, exogenous growth hormone—that is, growth hormone that isn't made by your own body—carries the risk of unwanted side effects. Blood sugar levels can increase to pre-diabetic levels. Blood pressure also goes up, and there is a theoretical increased risk of prostate cancer and heart problems. For these reasons, injections of artificial growth hormone are used rarely. But what if we could boost growth hormone naturally?

Meals very effectively suppress the secretion of growth hormone, so if we're eating three meals per day, we get effectively no growth hormone during the day. Worse, overeating suppresses growth hormone levels by as much as 80 percent.

The most potent natural stimulus to growth hormone secretion is fasting. In one study, over a five-day fasting period, growth hormone secretion more than doubled. During fasting, in addition to the usual early-morning spike of growth hormone (pulsatile), there is also regular secretion throughout the day (non-pulsatile). Both pulsatile and non-pulsatile release of growth hormone is increased during fasting. Interestingly, very low-calorie diets are not able to provoke the same growth hormone response.

A study of a religious forty-day fast found that baseline growth hormone levels increased from 0.73 ng/mL to peak at 9.86 ng/mL. That is a 1250 percent increase in growth hormone, all done without drugs. And a 1992 study showed a fivefold increase in growth hormone in response to a two-day fast.

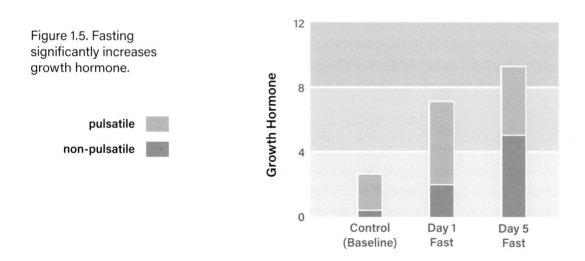

Figure 1.5. Fasting significantly increases growth hormone.

Source: Cahill, "Fuel Metabolism in Starvation."

BENEFITS FOR ATHLETES

All these hormonal changes may be particularly beneficial for athletes. First, their net physiological effect is to maintain lean mass (muscle and bone) over the fasting period, which has enormous implications for athletes. Second, while studies are few, the higher growth hormone level may improve recovery time from hard workouts. The increased adrenaline also allows a more intense workout. Athletes can train harder and recover faster. Many elite athletes are becoming more interested in the advantages of "training in the fasted state."

It is not by accident that many of the early proponents of training in the fasted state are bodybuilders. This is a sport that demands, in particular, high-intensity training and extremely low body fat. Brad Pilon, author of *Eat, Stop, Eat,* and Martin Berkhan, who popularized the LeanGains method of fasting, are both bodybuilders.

The Importance of Healthy Eating

Of course, fasting isn't a cure-all—healthy eating still matters.

Modern medicine's greatest challenges are metabolic diseases: obesity, type 2 diabetes, high blood pressure, high blood cholesterol, and fatty liver, collectively known as metabolic syndrome. The presence of any of these diseases tremendously increases the risk of heart disease, stroke, cancer, and premature death. And the roots of metabolic syndrome lie in the Western diet, with its abundance of sugar, high fructose corn syrup, artificial flavors, artificial sweeteners, and overdependence on refined grains.

Societies that have kept their traditional patterns of eating are not afflicted with these metabolic disorders. This book focuses on one particular facet of traditional eating patterns that is virtually forgotten in today's society: intermittent fasting. However, this is only part of the solution. For optimal health, it is not enough to simply add fasting to your life. You must also focus on healthy eating patterns.

What "healthy eating" doesn't mean

There is a tendency to define a healthy eating pattern as simply some combination of macronutrients. There are only three macronutrients: carbohydrates, proteins, and fats. Many "healthy" diets recommended by experts specify some percentage of these three—for example, the older *Dietary Guidelines for Americans* advised keeping dietary fat to less than 30 percent of total calories. The widespread adoption of nutrition and calorie labels on packaged food has unfortunately contributed to this view.

While this may appear scientific, there is no real basis for these recommendations. The underlying assumption of macronutrient-based guidelines is that all fats are equal, all carbohydrates are equal, and all proteins are equal. However, this is clearly false. Extra-virgin olive oil is not the same as trans-fat-laden margarine, even though both are pure fat. Our bodies respond completely differently to each one. Protein from wild salmon is not the same as highly refined gluten (which is a protein even though it's found in grains). Carbohydrates from sugar are not the same as carbohydrates from broccoli or kale. White bread is not the same as white beans. There are simple and easily measureable differences in the way our bodies metabolize these different foods.

The same holds true for calories. Dietary guidelines that specify calorie limits unwittingly assume that all calories are equal, but one hundred calories of a green salad does not have the fattening effect as one hundred calories of chocolate chip cookies.

Relying on macronutrient-based guidelines or calorie limits makes eating far more complicated than it should be. We do not eat a specific percentage of fats, protein, and carbohydrates. We eat foods. Certain foods are more fattening than others. Therefore, the best advice focuses on eating or not eating specific *foods*, not specific nutrients.

Because consistently high insulin levels are the root cause of all the diseases of metabolic syndrome, it's especially important for those with metabolic syndrome to consider how foods stimulate the release of insulin. Fasting, of course, is the ultimate weapon in your arsenal when it comes to lowering insulin levels—since all foods stimulate insulin to some degree, the best way to lower insulin is to eat nothing at all. However, we cannot fast indefinitely, so there are some simple rules to follow to lower insulin levels.

Eat whole, unprocessed foods

Humans evolved to eat a wide range of foods without detrimental health consequences. The Inuit peoples traditionally ate diets extremely high in animal products, which means high percentages of fat and protein. Others, such as the Okinawans, ate a traditional diet based on root vegetables, which means it's high in carbohydrates. But both populations traditionally did not suffer metabolic diseases. These only appeared with the increasing Westernization of their diets.

What humans *haven't* evolved to eat are highly processed foods. During processing, the natural balance of macronutrients, fiber, and micronutrients is completely disrupted. For example, processing the wheat berry to remove all the fat and protein means that the result, white flour, is almost pure carbohydrates. Wheat berries are natural; white flour is not. It is also ground to an extremely fine consistency that greatly speeds the absorption of carbohydrates into the bloodstream. Most other processed grains suffer the same problems. Our body has evolved to handle natural foods, and when we feed it unnatural ones, the result is illness.

Imagine a beautiful red Ferrari sports car sitting in the driveway. Then imagine that we "process" it by removing the doors and wheels and adding bicycle tires and rusty blue doors from a truck. Is it the same car? Not at all.

There is nothing inherently unhealthy about carbohydrate-containing foods. The problem arises when we start changing these foods from their natural state and then consuming them in large amounts. The same also applies to processed fats. Processing transforms relatively innocuous vegetable oils into fats that contain trans fats, toxins whose dangers have now been well recognized.

Foods should be recognizable in their natural state as something that was alive or has come out of the ground. Boxes of Cheerios do not grow in the ground. If it comes prepackaged in a bag or a box, it should be avoided. If it has a nutrition label, it should be avoided. Real foods, whether broccoli or beef, have no labels.

The true secret to healthy eating is this: Just eat real food.

Reduce sugars and refined grains

Avoiding all processed foods is preferable but not always 100 percent possible, for many reasons. It is therefore important to recognize which foods are the biggest offenders, so that we may avoid them.

For everyone, but especially for those with metabolic syndrome, it's most important to avoid sugars and refined grains, such as flour and corn products. These are more fattening than other foods, even when they contain the same number of calories, which is why low-carbohydrate diets are effective for weight loss.

Eat more natural fats

For many decades, dietary fat was considered public enemy number one. (We'll talk more about the misconceptions behind low-fat diets for weight loss in Chapter 5 and for heart health in Chapter 8.) Gradually, health authorities have come to recognize that it has been unfairly targeted. In fact, although the term *healthy fats* was once considered an oxymoron, they're now just a well-accepted fact of life. Foods high in monounsaturated fats, such as olive oil, nuts, and avocados, which were previously shunned, are now considered "superfoods" because they are so healthy. Consuming fatty fish, such as wild salmon, has been proven to reduce the risk of heart disease. And more and more evidence is showing that naturally occurring saturated fats, such as those found in meat and dairy, are also not harmful to our health.

Eat less artificial fats

But not all fats are so innocent. Partially hydrogenated vegetable oils—found in foods such as shortening, deep-fried foods, margarine, and baked goods such as cakes and cookies—contain trans fats, which our bodies do not handle well. Trans fats raise LDL ("bad") cholesterol and lower HDL ("good") cholesterol, increasing the risk of heart disease and stroke.

Highly processed vegetable oils, such as corn, sunflower, and canola oils, were once considered "heart healthy." It's easy to mistake corn oil, for instance, for a natural fat. But actually, corn is not naturally oily. To fill the bottle of corn oil you can buy so cheaply in the supermarket requires processing literally tons of corn. And as it turns out, recent data suggests that these oils are very high in inflammatory omega-6 fats. While some omega-6 fats are necessary, we are likely eating ten to twenty times more than we did in the past, and when our consumption of omega-6 fats is out of balance with our consumption of omega-3 fats (found in fatty cold-water fish, nuts, and seeds), the result is systemic inflammation, which is a factor in heart disease, type 2 diabetes, inflammatory bowel disease, and other chronic illnesses.

Eating more healthy fats and avoiding artificial fats, such as partially hydrogenated oils and highly processed vegetable oils, is key for good health.

> **The basics of good nutrition can be summarized in these simple rules.**
> **Eat whole, unprocessed foods.**
> **Avoid sugar.**
> **Avoid refined grains.**
> **Eat a diet high in natural fats.**
> **Balance feeding with fasting.**

Different Kinds of Fasting

There are many different ways to fast, and there is no one "correct" way to do it. An absolute fast withholds both food and liquid. This may be done for religious purposes, such as during the holy month of Ramadan in the Muslim tradition. During that time, no food or drink is consumed during the period between sunrise and sunset.

Medically, this combines the food restriction of fasting with dehydration due to the restriction of fluids. This makes an absolute fast much more physically difficult and limits the duration to fairly short periods. Absolute fasts are not generally recommended for health purposes. The accompanying dehydration confers no additional health benefits that compensate for the increase in difficulty. The risk of medical complications is also much higher with absolute fasts.

We will cover many different fasting schedules later in the book. Intermittent fasting can be successfully implemented with either short fasts (less than twenty-four hours) or longer fasts (more than twenty-four hours). Extended fasting (more than three days) can also be safely used for weight loss and other health benefits.

We'll explain in detail the "best practices" for fasting in Chapter 10, but in general, we encourage consuming plenty of noncaloric liquids (water, tea, coffee) and homemade bone broth, which is full of nutrients.

Overall Effects of Fasting

What about potential side effects of fasting? Increased glucose? Nope. Increased blood pressure? Nope. Higher risk of cancer? Nope. Actually, fasting has the opposite effects—lower glucose, lower blood pressure, and lower risk of cancer. Plus, we reap all the benefits of the increased growth hormone.

Fasting does not make you tired. Fasting does not burn muscle. There is no starvation mode from fasting where you shrivel up into the fetal position on your couch.

Rather, fasting has the potential to unleash the anti-aging properties of growth hormone without any of the problems of taking artificial growth hormone. In future chapters, we'll look in depth at how fasting helps with weight loss (Chapter 5) and type 2 diabetes (Chapter 6), boosts brainpower and slows aging (Chapter 7), and improves heart health (Chapter 8). All of these benefits are achieved without drugs, supplements, or any costs.

References

A. S. Cornford, A. L. Barkan, and J. F. Horowitz, "Rapid Suppression of Growth Hormone Concentration by Overeating: Potential Mediation by Hyperinsulinemia," *Journal of Clinical Endocrinology and Metabolism* 96, no. 3 (2011): 824–30.

Barry M. Popkin and Kiyah J. Duffey, "Does Hunger and Satiety Drive Eating Anymore?: Increasing Eating Occasions and Decreasing Time Between Eating Occasions in the United States," *American Journal of Clinical Nutrition* 91, no. 5 (2010): 1342–7.

Christian Zauner, Bruno Schneeweiss, Alexander Kranz, Christian Madl, Klaus Ratheiser, Ludwig Kramer, Erich Roth, Barbara Schneider, and Kurt Lenz, "Resting Energy Expenditure in Short-Term Starvation Is Increased as a Result of an Increase in Serum Norepinephrine," *American Journal of Clinical Nutrition* 71, no. 6 (2000): 1511–5.

Daniel Rudman, Axel G. Feller, Hoskote S. Nagraj, Gregory A. Gergans, Pardee Y. Lalitha, Allen F. Goldberg, Robert A. Schlenker, Lester Cohn, Inge W. Rudman, and Dale E. Mattson, "Effects of Human Growth Hormone in Men over 60 Years Old," *New England Journal of Medicine* 323 (1990): 1–6.

Ernst J. Drenick, Marion E. Swendseid, William H. Blahd, and Stewart G. Tuttle, "Prolonged Starvation as Treatment for Severe Obesity," *JAMA* 187, no. 2 (1964): 100–05.

George F. Cahill Jr., "Fuel Metabolism in Starvation," *Annual Review of Nutrition* 26 (2006): 1–22.

Helene Nørrelund, Anne Lene Riis, and Niels Møller, "Effects of GH on Protein Metabolism During Dietary Restriction in Man," *Growth Hormone & IGF Research* 12, no. 4 (2002): 198–207.

Helene Nørrelund, K. Sreekumaran Nair, Jens Otto Lunde Jørgensen, Jens Sandahl Christiansen, and Niels Møller, "The Protein-Retaining Effects of Growth Hormone During Fasting Involve Inhibition of Muscle-Protein Breakdown," *Diabetes* 50, no. 1 (2001): 96–104.

J. Oscarsson, M. Ottosson, and S. Eden, "Effects of Growth Hormone on Lipoprotein Lipase and Hepatic Lipase," *Journal of Endocrinological Investigation* 22 (1999): 2–9.

K. Y. Ho, J. D. Veldhuis, M. L. Johnson, R. Furlanetto, W. S. Evans, K. G. Alberti, and M. O. Thorner, "Fasting Enhances Growth Hormone Secretion and Amplifies the Complex Rhythms of Growth Hormone Secretion in Man," *Journal of Clinical Investigation* 81, no. 4 (1988): 968–75.

Mary Lee Vance, "Can Growth Hormone Prevent Aging?" *New England Journal of Medicine* 348 (2003): 779–80.

M. L. Hartman, J. D. Veldhuis, M. L. Johnson, M. M. Lee, K. G. Alberti, E. Samojlik, and M. O. Thorner, "Augmented Growth Hormone (GH) Secretory Burst Frequency and Amplitude Mediate Enhanced GH Secretion During a Two-Day Fast in Normal Men," *Journal of Clinical Endocrinology and Metabolism* 74, no. 4 (1992): 757–65.

M. R. Blackman, J. D. Sorkin, T. Münzer, M. F. Bellantoni, J. Busby-Whitehead, T. E. Stevens, J. Jayme, et al., "Growth Hormone and Sex Steroid Administration in Healthy Aged Women and Men: A Randomized Controlled Trial," *JAMA* 288, no. 18 (2002): 2282–92

Peter R. Kerndt, James L. Naughton, Charles E. Driscoll, and David A. Loxtercamp, "Fasting: The History, Pathophysiology and Complications," *Western Journal of Medicine* 137 (1982): 379–99.

S. Klein, O. B. Holland, and R. R. Wolfe, "Importance of Blood Glucose Concentration in Regulating Lipolysis During Fasting in Humans," *American Journal of Physiology—Endocrinology and Metabolism* 258, no. 1 (1990): E32–E39.

W. K. Stewart and Laura W. Fleming, "Features of a Successful Therapeutic Fast of 382 Days' Duration," *Postgraduate Medical Journal* 49 (1973): 203–9.

SAMANTHA

FASTING SUCCESS STORY

In 1999, I was diagnosed with polycystic ovary syndrome (PCOS), a condition associated with insulin resistance that also includes other horrible symptoms such as weight gain, hirsutism, a skin condition called acanthosis nigricans, and early development of diabetes. I tried lots of things to fix my PCOS—natural herbs, progesterone therapy, and so on. Nothing worked.

In May 2015, when I was thirty-seven, I was also diagnosed with type 2 diabetes. I had been trying to prevent this, and here it was anyway. My grandmother had suffered with it for years and experienced massive blood clots and loss of the use of her hands and eyes, and she eventually died from its complications. My mother-in-law died from a diabetes-related heart attack at age sixty-two. Two elderly neighbors had lost their legs to it. I already knew diabetes is evil and unmerciful. It steals from you every day, makes your life miserable, and then kills you. I figured I'd be dead by sixty, maybe seventy if I was lucky.

My doctor didn't give me any hope, either. She said, "Diabetes is a progressive disease. The medication I'm going to prescribe you will help delay the consequences of having diabetes for about ten years, but after that, you will develop some or all of these symptoms: loss of your eyesight, loss of the use of your legs and/or feet, or possibly loss of those limbs entirely, loss of sensation in your hands, high blood pressure, which could result in stroke or heart attack, pain in different areas of your body . . . " I asked her if I could resolve this with diet and exercise. In response, she just repeated, "Diabetes is a progressive disease."

I was just looking for any hope, even a slim chance that I could beat this. Instead, she gave me four prescriptions to treat my diabetes, high blood pressure, and high cholesterol. But I had no intention of taking any medication. I knew one thing for sure: everyone I knew who'd got on diabetes medication had lived miserably and eventually died from the disease.

I spent several hours that night researching on the Internet, and I discovered Dr. Jason Fung. He was the only person, let alone doctor, that I found who not only advocated a diet change but pinpointed fasting as the key.

I started immediately on a water-only fasting regimen. I used mostly three- to five-day fasts because I wanted quick results that I couldn't undo by eating something wrong. I wasn't focused on weight loss but on beating diabetes—still, I lost twelve pounds the first month and then six pounds a month thereafter, for thirty pounds in four months—I went from 256 pounds to 226. Although alternate-day fasting doesn't slow your metabolism, multiple-day fasts do seem to slow it a little. But the improvement in insulin sensitivity is well worth a long fast over a short one.

In addition to fasting regularly, I changed my diet. Dr. Fung supports any whole-food approach that limits processed foods in addition to fasting, without dictating which diet is best. I chose to do low-carb. Previously, everything I ate was underpinned with rice or pasta. Now I learned that meat and vegetables alone are fine. I underpin my foods with bulgur wheat, finely chopped and sautéed cauliflower, spaghetti squash, or just well-buttered and seasoned vegetables. I try to mix cheese and nuts into every meal because they fill me up. I even learned how to make sweet and spicy hot wings using hot sauce, balsamic vinegar, xylitol, and oil from the renderings from baking the wings.

For the first month on my fasting regimen, I took a multivitamin, magnesium, B-complex vitamin, and vitamin D every day. For the second month, I used only magnesium, a B-complex vitamin, potassium, and Himalayan pink salt. It helped reduce the coldness in my feet and hands for some reason. I started supplementing with 500 to 1000 mcg of chromium per day starting in month 3. It really helped me to get my blood sugars to fall to preprandial levels within two hours of eating a meal instead of four hours. In September 2015, four months after I was diagnosed with type 2 diabetes and began my fasting regimen, I got a blood sugar reading in the 70s for the first time ever. This reading was so unusual for me that I had to go back and look up what was normal!

I wasn't expecting it, but fasting also resolved the PCOS. The fact is, I have not been this healthy—ever! Even when I was twenty years old in the military and had 21 percent body fat, running three to five miles per day, five days per week, I was not this healthy.

Here's what happened symptom by symptom:

Immediately after I started fasting, the tingling, numbness, swelling, and burning in my left foot went away. A burning in my left upper thigh near my hip took longer to go away, but after four months I had complete relief. My fingers used to go to sleep, and now that happens rarely and is limited to only my left pinky finger.

I suffered from chronic yeast and bacterial infections, which are now gone completely. The hair on my face from the PCOS-related hirsutism is disappearing, and what's left is finer and softer. The hair on my head is softer and naturally oiled instead of dry and flaking. I have a smaller waistline and a nicer butt—so says my husband! My period has returned on time each month, starting at the beginning of July, just two months after I began the fasting regimen.

My blood pressure dropped from 142/92 to 128/83 in one month. By September, it was 101/75—without any medication. The prescriptions the doctor sent me are still in the envelopes.

Chapter 2
A BRIEF HISTORY OF FASTING ▮▮▮▮▮

There is nothing new, except what has been forgotten.

—Marie Antoinette

From an evolutionary standpoint, eating three meals a day and snacking throughout the day is not a requirement for survival or good health. Before the modern era, food availability was unpredictable and highly irregular. Drought, war, insect infestations, and disease all played a part in restricting food, sometimes to the point of starvation. So did the seasons: during the summer and fall, fruits and vegetables were plentiful, but during the winter and spring, they were scarce. Periods without food could last weeks or even months. There's a reason that one of the Four Horsemen of the Apocalypse is Famine.

As human societies developed agriculture, these periods of famine were gradually reduced and eventually eliminated. However, ancient civilizations, like the Greeks, recognized there was something deeply, intrinsically beneficial to periodic fasting. As periods of involuntary starvation faded, ancient cultures replaced them with periods of voluntary fasting. These were often called times of "cleansing," "detoxification," or "purification." The earliest recorded histories of ancient Greece show an unyielding belief in their power. Indeed, fasting is the most time-honored and widespread healing tradition in the world. It has been practiced by virtually every culture and every religion on earth. Fasting is an ancient, time-tested tradition.

Spiritual Fasting

Fasting is widely practiced for spiritual purposes and remains part of virtually every major religion in the world. Three of the most influential men in the history of the world, Jesus Christ, Buddha, and the Prophet Muhammad all shared a common belief in the healing power of fasting. In spiritual terms, it is often called cleansing or purification, but practically, it amounts to the same thing.

The practice of fasting developed independently among different religions and cultures, not as something that was harmful but as something that was deeply, intrinsically beneficial to the human body and spirit. Fasting is not so much a treatment for illness but a treatment for *wellness*. The regular application of fasting helps protect people from illness and keeps them feeling well.

In the story of Adam and Eve, the only act that is prohibited in the Garden of Eden is to eat the fruit of one tree, and Eve is tempted by the serpent to betray this trust. Fasting is thus an act of turning away from temptation and back toward God.

In the Bible, Matthew 4:2 states, "Then Jesus was led by the Spirit into the wilderness to be tempted by the devil. After fasting forty days and forty nights, he was hungry." (I'll mention here the interesting point that hunger often disappears during extended fasts, which has been noted throughout history.) In the Christian

One unexpected consequence of fasting is the feeling of a strong connection with my ancient ancestors and in particular my cavewoman ancestor for whom fasting was an everyday, normal reality. She, and all the subsequent ancient ancestors, not only survived but were likely to have been extremely healthy and strong. I think of them with great fondness and affection. Going without food for long stretches is what we evolved to do.

—Stella B., Leeds, UK

For millions of people across the world, regular fasting is commonplace and has been part of spiritual practice for thousands of years. But before that, fasting was simply a way of life. With no storable grains, and few other foods that stayed fresh for very long, most of our ancestors experienced both feast and famine on a regular basis. When game was scarce, seasons changed, or the pickings were slim, hunter-gatherers did without. Eating all the time is not normal.

tradition, fasting and prayer are often methods of cleansing and renewing the soul. Symbolically, believers empty their souls so that they may be ready to receive God. Fasting is not so much about self-denial but about a reaching for spirituality and being able to commune with God and hear his voice. By fasting, you put your body under submission to the Holy Spirit, humble your soul before the presence of God, and prepare yourself to hear the voice of God.

Greek Orthodox Christians may follow various fasts on 180 to 200 days of the year. Famous nutrition researcher Ancel Keys often considered Crete the poster child for the healthy Mediterranean diet. However, there was a critically important factor of their diet that he completely dismissed: most of the population of Crete followed the Greek Orthodox tradition of fasting. This may have contributed to the healthy longevity of this population.

Buddhist monks are known to abstain from eating after noon, fasting until the next morning. In addition, there may be water-only fasts for days or weeks on end. They fast to quench their human desires, which helps them rise above all desires in order to achieve nirvana and end all suffering. This fits with their core beliefs in moderation and austerity.

Hinduism embraces fasting in the belief that our sins lessen as the body suffers. It is also seen as a method of cultivating control over desires and guiding the mind toward peace: the physical needs of the body are denied for spiritual gains. Certain days of the week are designated for fasting in Hinduism, as are certain days of the month. Fasting is also common at festivals. Traditional

Ayurvedic medicine also ascribes the cause of many illnesses to the accumulation of toxins in the body and prescribes fasting to cleanse these toxins.

Muslims fast from sunrise to sunset during the holy month of Ramadan. According to the Qur'an, the Prophet Muhammad said, "The month of Ramadan is a blessed month, a month in which Allah has made fasting obligatory." The Prophet Muhammad also encouraged fasting on Mondays and Thursdays. Ramadan is the best studied of the fasting periods, but it differs from many fasting protocols in that fluids are forbidden, which results in a period of mild dehydration.

The Early Adopters

One early fasting advocate was Hippocrates of Cos (c. 460–c. 370 BC), widely considered the father of modern medicine. In his lifetime, people came to the realization that obesity was an evolving and serious disease. Hippocrates wrote, "Sudden death is more common in those who are naturally fat than in the lean." He advised that treatment for obesity should include exertion after meals and eating a high-fat diet, and he recommended that "they should, moreover, eat only once a day." In other words, incorporating a daily twenty-four-hour fast was even then recognized as highly beneficial in the treatment of obesity. Proving once again that Hippocrates is worthy of our reverence, he also recognized the benefits of physical exercise and eating plenty of healthy fats in a healthy lifestyle.

The ancient Greek writer and historian Plutarch (c. 46–c. 120) echoed these sentiments. He wrote, "Instead of using medicine, better fast today." Renowned ancient Greek thinkers Plato and his student Aristotle were also staunch supporters of fasting.

The ancient Greeks believed that medical treatments could be observed from nature, and since humans, like most animals, naturally avoid eating when they become sick, they believed fasting to be a natural remedy for illness. In fact, fasting can be considered an instinct, since all animals—dogs, cats, cattle, sheep, and also humans—avoid food when sick. Think about the last time you had the flu, or even a cold. The last thing you probably wanted to do was eat. So fasting can be considered a universal human instinct for handling multiple kinds of illnesses. It's truly ingrained in human heritage, and it's as old as mankind itself.

The ancient Greeks also believed that fasting improved mental and cognitive abilities, and they recognized that they could solve problems and puzzles better during fasting. This is easy to understand. Think about the last time you ate a huge Thanksgiving meal. Did you feel more energetic and mentally alert afterwards? Or did you feel sleepy and a little dopey? Most of us feel sleepy. After a large meal, blood is shunted to your digestive system to cope with the huge influx of food, leaving less blood to go to the brain. The result? A food coma. Maybe a little nap. Now think about a time when you had not eaten for many hours. Do you remember being lethargic and mentally sluggish? Not likely. It is more likely you felt mentally sharp and completely attuned to your environment. This is not by accident. In Paleolithic times, we needed all our mental faculties and keen senses to find food. When food was scarce, our alertness and mental focus naturally increased.

Other intellectual giants throughout history were also great proponents of fasting. Paracelsus (1493–1541), a Swiss German physician and the founder of toxicology, famously wrote, "The dose makes the poison." He critically observed nature and laid the groundwork for modern scientific methods. His discoveries revolutionized medicine. As a military surgeon, he rejected the old practices of applying cow dung to wounds and instead insisted they be kept clean and protected. He also objected to the common medical practice of bloodletting. Instead of following these common practices, he pioneered clinical diagnosis and application of specific treatments. A brilliant and transformative scientist, he also wrote, "Fasting is the greatest remedy—the physician within."

Benjamin Franklin (1706–1790), one of America's founding fathers, was world-renowned for his extensive knowledge in a wide range of areas. He was a leading scientist, inventor, diplomat, and author. Turning his genius to medicine, he once wrote, "The best of all medicines is resting and fasting."

And finally, Mark Twain (1835–1910), one of America's foremost writers and philosophers, once wrote, "A little starvation can really do more for the average sick man than can the best medicines and the best doctors."

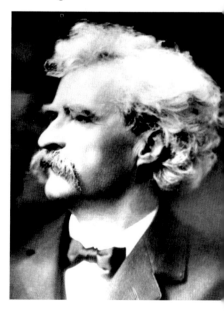

Mark Twain was an advocate of fasting for health.

Modern Fasting

Interestingly, in the late 1800s and early 1900s, professional fasters would fast for entertainment. One fasted for thirty days and drank a quantity of his own urine. (Talk about being starved for entertainment!) Franz Kafka based his short story "A Hunger Artist" on the practice. The fad soon died out, never to be reborn. My guess is that watching someone not eat really is not that entertaining.

Fasting began to appear in the medical literature in the early 1900s. In 1915, an article in the *Journal of Biological Chemistry* described fasting as "a perfectly safe, harmless, and effective method for reducing the weight of those suffering from obesity." However, in a time rife with poverty, infectious diseases, and war, obesity was hardly the problem it is today. Severe food shortages were present during the two world wars and the intervening Great Depression. Treatments for obesity were not a priority.

In the late 1950s, Dr. W. L. Bloom reignited interest in short-term fasting as a therapeutic measure, but longer periods were also well described in the literature. In a study published in 1968, Dr. I. C. Gilliland reported his experience with forty-six patients "whose reducing regime started with a standard absolute fast for 14 days."

After the late 1960s, interest in therapeutic fasting seemed to again fade, mostly because obesity was still not a major public health issue. Coronary heart disease was the major health concern of the time, and nutritional research focused on dietary fat and cholesterol. Commercial interests also became pervasive, and as you might guess, large food corporations will not support any intervention that threatens their existence. So fasting as an adjunct to diet started to fade. Despite the fact that fasting is low-fat, as well as low-everything-else, it had almost entirely disappeared by the 1980s.

For most of human history, large amounts of food were not readily accessible all throughout the day. Intermittent fasting was likely a regular part of human evolution, and it's possible our bodies—and brains—have come to expect periods of food scarcity.

Because we are blessed with abundant food all year round in the twenty-first century, we now have to make a special effort to *impose* food scarcity upon ourselves for therapeutic purposes.

Despite its long traditions, advantages, and effectiveness, fasting as a therapeutic tool has been extinct for the last thirty-plus years. Even its very mention tends to bring ridicule. But, in truth, the idea is very straightforward. If metabolic diseases such as type 2 diabetes are caused by eating too much, then logically, the solution is to eat little to balance it out. What could be simpler?

References

Christos S. Mantzoros, ed., *Obesity and Diabetes* (Totowa, NJ: Humana Press, 2006).

Hippocrates, *Hippocratic Writings*, ed. G. E. R. Lloyd (New York: Penguin Classics, 1983).

I. C. Gilliland, "Total Fasting in the Treatment of Obesity," *Postgraduate Medical Journal* 44, no. 507 (1968): 58–61.

Otto Folin and W. Denis, "On Starvation and Obesity, with Special Reference to Acidosis," *Journal of Biological Chemistry* 21 (1915): 183–192.

Chapter 3
BUSTING THE MYTHS OF FASTING

Although fasting was widely practiced historically, most of us today grew up believing some fundamental myths about the dangers of fasting. They are repeated so often that they are often perceived as infallible truths. Some of the more common myths include:

> Fasting puts you in "starvation mode"
>
> Fasting makes you burn muscle
>
> Fasting causes low blood sugar
>
> Fasting results in overeating
>
> Fasting deprives the body of nutrients
>
> "It's just crazy"

Although they were long ago disproven, these myths still persist. Most people mistakenly believe fasting is detrimental to health. The truth is quite the opposite—there are a significant number of health benefits, as we'll explore in later chapters. But first, let's examine these myths.

Myth #1: Fasting Puts You in "Starvation Mode"

"Starvation mode" is the mysterious bogeyman always raised to scare us away from missing even a single meal. Why is it so bad to skip a meal? Let's get some perspective here. Assuming we eat three meals per day, over one year, that's a little over a thousand meals. To think that fasting for one day, skipping three meals of the one thousand, will somehow cause irreparable harm is simply absurd.

The idea of "starvation mode" refers to the notion that our metabolism decreases severely and our bodies "shut down" in response to fasting. We can test this notion by looking at the basal metabolic rate (BMR), which measures the amount of energy that our body burns in order to function normally—to keep the lungs breathing, brain functioning, heart pumping, kidneys, liver, and digestive system all working, and so on. Most of the calories we spend each day are not used for exercise but for these basic functions.

The BMR is not a fixed number but actually increases or decreases up to 40 percent in response to many variables. For example, I never seemed to get cold as a teenager. Even skiing in -22°F weather, I stayed warm. My BMR was high—I was burning a lot of calories to keep my body temperature up. As I've gotten older, I've noticed that I no longer endure the cold so well. I also eat far less than I did as a teenager. My BMR has gotten lower, so I no longer burn as many calories on basic body functions. This is what most people mean when they say that metabolism slows down with age, and it contributes to the well-known tendency of older "snowbirds" from the Northeast and Canada to retire in warm places like Florida and Arizona.

Daily caloric reduction has been well documented to cause a dramatic reduction in BMR. In studies with a baseline daily calorie consumption of approximately 2500 calories per day, reducing calories consumed to approximately 1500 calories a day for a long stretch of time will result in a 25 to 30 percent reduction in BMR. On the other hand, overfeeding studies, where subjects are asked to deliberately eat more than they normally do, causes an increase in BMR.

Reduced metabolism makes us generally cold, tired, hungry, and less energetic—our bodies are essentially conserving energy by not burning calories to keep us warm and moving. From a weight standpoint, reduced metabolism is a double curse. First, we feel lousy while dieting. Even worse, because we're burning fewer calories per day, it's both harder to lose weight and much easier to gain weight back after we've lost it. This is the main problem with most caloric-reduction diets.

Suppose you normally eat 2000 calories a day and cut back to only 1500. Your body cannot run a deficit indefinitely—it will eventually run out of fat to burn—so it plans ahead and decreases your energy expenditure. The end result is a decreased BMR. This has been proven repeatedly by experiments over the last century, and we'll talk about it in more detail in Chapter 5. Because of this well-known "starvation mode" effect of daily caloric restriction, many people assume that fasting will result in a similar but more severe decrease in BMR.

Luckily, this does not happen. If short-term fasting dropped our metabolism, humans as a species would not likely have survived. Consider the situation of repeated feast/famine cycles. During long winters back in the Paleolithic era, there were many days where no food was available. After the first episode, you would be severely weakened as your metabolism falls. After several repeated episodes, you would be so weak that you would be unable to hunt or gather food, making you even weaker. This is a vicious cycle that the human species would not have survived. Our bodies do not shut down in response to short-term fasting.

In fact, metabolism revs *up*, not down, during fasting. This makes sense from a survival standpoint. If we do not eat, our bodies use our stored energy as fuel so that we can find more food. Humans have not evolved to *require* three meals a day, every day.

When food intake goes to zero (fasting), our body obviously cannot take BMR down to zero—we have to burn *some* calories just to stay alive. Instead, hormones allow the body to switch energy sources from food to body fat. After all, that is precisely why we carry body fat—to be used for food when no food is available. It's not there for looks. By "feeding" on our own fat, we significantly increase the availability of "food," and this is matched by an increase in energy expenditure.

Studies demonstrate this phenomenon clearly. In one, fasting every other day for twenty-two days resulted in no measurable decrease in BMR. There was no starvation mode. Fat oxidation—fat burning—increased 58 percent, from 64 g/day to 101 g/day. Carbohydrate oxidation decreased 53 percent, from 175 g/day to 81 g/day. This means that the body has started to switch over from burning sugar to burning fat, with no overall drop in energy.

In another study, four days of continuous fasting *increased* BMR by 12 percent. Levels of the neurotransmitter norepinephrine (also known as noradrenaline), which prepares the body for action, increased by 117 percent, keeping energy levels high. Fatty acids in the bloodstream increased over 370 percent as the body switched over from burning food to burning stored fats.

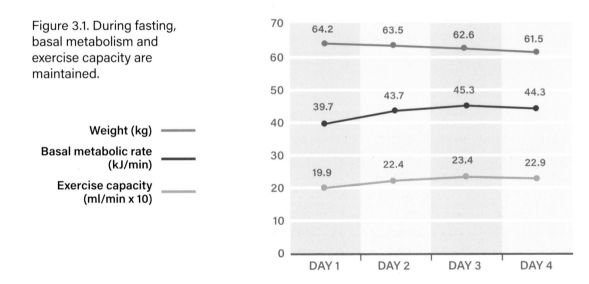

Figure 3.1. During fasting, basal metabolism and exercise capacity are maintained.

Weight (kg) ——

Basal metabolic rate (kJ/min) ——

Exercise capacity (ml/min x 10) ——

Source: Zauner et al., "Resting Energy Expenditure in Short-Term Starvation Is Increased as a Result of an Increase in Serum Norepinephrine."

The "fasting is unhealthy" reflex is largely an outcome of the marketing push to encourage consumers to buy food. An enormous amount of advertising money is spent every year in an effort to convince consumers that at any moment that they are not consuming food, they are at risk for underperforming. The Snickers campaign launched in 2015 offers a perfect example: candy bars labeled with words—"sleepy," "grouchy," "impatient," etc. —hinted that these undesirable conditions were best overcome by consuming food, essentially claiming psychoactive effects for the candy bar.

We'll explore how the body stores energy and accesses it in more detail in Chapter 5, but for now, just know that we're designed to function well during periods of fasting—our bodies don't start to shut down or go into "starvation mode."

Myth #2: Fasting Makes You Burn Muscle

One persistent myth of fasting is that it burns muscle, that our body, if we're not eating, will immediately start using our muscles as an energy source. This does not actually happen.

The human body evolved to survive periods of fasting. We store food energy as body fat and use this as fuel when food is not available. Muscle, on the other hand, is preserved until body fat becomes so low that the body has no choice but to turn to muscle. This will only happen when body fat is at less than 4 percent. (For comparison, elite male marathon runners carry approximately 8 percent body fat and female marathoners slightly more.) If we did not preserve muscle and burn fat instead when no food is available, we would not have survived very long as a species. Almost all mammals have this same ability.

Real-world studies of fasting show that the concern over muscle loss is largely misplaced. Alternate-day fasting over

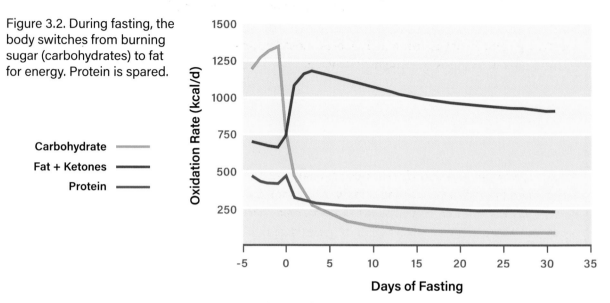

Figure 3.2. During fasting, the body switches from burning sugar (carbohydrates) to fat for energy. Protein is spared.

Carbohydrate ————
Fat + Ketones ————
Protein ————

Oxidation Rate (kcal/d)

Days of Fasting

Source: McCue, ed., *Comparative Physiology of Fasting, Starvation, and Food Limitation.*

seventy days decreased body weight by 6 percent, but fat mass decreased by 11.4 percent and lean mass (muscle and bone) did not change at all.

At baseline, eating normally, energy comes from a mix of carbohydrates, fat, and protein. As you start fasting, the body increases carbohydrate oxidation. This is just a fancy way of saying that it is burning sugar, in the form of glycogen, for the first twenty-four to forty-eight hours after you stop eating, until it runs out of glycogen. With no more sugar to burn, the body switches to burning fat. Fat oxidation increases as carbohydrate oxidation decreases toward zero. (See Figure 3.2.)

At the same time, protein oxidation—that is, burning protein, such as muscle, for fuel—actually *decreases.* The normal protein breakdown of around seventy-five grams per day falls to fifteen to twenty grams per day during fasting. Rather than burning muscle during fasting, we start *conserving* muscle. Much of the amino acids that are broken down during regular turnover of cells are reabsorbed into new proteins.

Running just on the fat stored in their bodies, most Americans could walk from New York to Florida without technically needing a bite to eat.

After all, why would your body store excess energy as fat if it meant to burn protein as soon as the chips were down? Muscles and other proteins are functional tissues and have many purposes. They are not designed to store energy. Glycogen and fat are. To burn muscle for energy would be like storing firewood and then, as soon as cold weather hits, chopping up your sofa and throwing it into the fire.

In fact, fasting is one of the most potent stimuli for growth hormone secretion, and increased growth hormone helps maintain lean body mass. In studies that used drugs to suppress growth hormone in fasted subjects, there was a 50 percent increase in protein oxidation.

Muscle gain or loss is mostly a function of exercise. You can't eat your way to more muscle. Supplement companies, of course, try to convince you otherwise. Taking creatine and drinking whey protein shakes do not build muscle. That's wishful thinking. Exercise is the only reliable way to build muscle.

If you are worried about muscle loss, exercise more. It's not rocket science. Diet and exercise are two entirely separate issues. Don't confuse the two. Don't worry about what your diet (or lack of diet—that is, fasting) is doing to your muscle mass. Exercise builds muscle. Lack of exercise leads to atrophy of muscles.

On the other hand, if you are worried about weight loss and type 2 diabetes, then you need to worry about diet, not exercise. You can't outrun a bad diet.

So let me lay it out as simply as I can. Body fat is, at its core, stored energy for us to "eat" when there is no food. It's not there for looks, right? So, when we fast, we "eat" our own fat. This is natural.

Figure 3.3. There was no loss of fat-free mass during 70 days of alternate-day fasting.

	Baseline	Alternate-Day Fasting
	Day 1	Day 70
Body weight (kg)	96.4 ± 5.3	90.8 ± 4.8
BMI (kg/m²)	33.7 ± 1.0	31.4 ± 0.9
Fat mass (kg)	43.0 ± 2.2	38.1 ± 1.8
Fat-free mass (kg)	52.0 ± 3.6	51.9 ± 3.7
Waist circumference (cm)	109 ± 2	105 ± 3

Source: Bhutani et al., "Improvements in Coronary Heart Disease Risk Indicators by Alternate-Day Fasting Involve Adipose Tissue Modulations."

This is normal. This is the way we were designed. Otherwise, famine cycles in Paleolithic times would have eventually left us as a ball of 100 percent fat! During fasting, hormonal changes kick in to give us more energy (increased adrenaline) and preserve our lean muscles and bones (increased growth hormone). This is normal and natural and there is nothing here to be feared.

Myth #3: Fasting Causes Low Blood Sugar

Sometimes people worry that blood sugar will fall very low during fasting and they will become shaky and sweaty. Luckily, this does not actually happen. Blood sugar level is tightly monitored by the body, and there are multiple mechanisms to keep it in the proper range. During fasting, our body begins by breaking down glycogen (remember, that's the glucose in short-term storage) in the liver to provide glucose. This happens every night as you sleep to keep blood sugars normal as you fast overnight.

People who engage in fasting for religious or spiritual purposes often report feelings of extreme clear-headedness and physical and emotional well-being. Some even feel a sense of euphoria. They usually attribute this to achieving some kind of spiritual enlightenment, but the truth is much more down-to-earth and scientific than that: *it's* *the ketones!* Ketones are a "superfood" for the brain. When the body and brain are fueled primarily by fatty acids and ketones, respectively, the "brain fog," mood swings, and emotional instability that are caused by wild fluctuations in blood sugar become a thing of the past and clear thinking is the new normal.

If you fast for longer than twenty-four to thirty-six hours, glycogen stores become depleted. The liver now can manufacture new glucose in a process called gluconeogenesis, using the glycerol that's a by-product of the breakdown of fat. This means that we do not need to eat glucose for our blood glucose levels to remain normal.

A related myth is that brain cells can only use glucose for energy. This is incorrect. Human brains, unique amongst animals, can also use ketone bodies—particles that are produced when fat is metabolized—as a fuel source. This allows us to function optimally even when food is not readily available. Ketones provide the majority of the energy we need.

Consider the consequences if glucose were absolutely necessary for brain function. After twenty-four hours without food, glucose stored in our bodies in the form of glycogen is depleted. At that point, we'd become blubbering idiots as our brains shut down. In the Paleolithic era, our intellect was our only advantage against wild animals with their sharp claws, sharp fangs, and bulging muscles. Without it, humans would have become extinct long ago.

When glucose is not available, the body begins to burn fat and produce ketone bodies, which are able to cross the blood-brain barrier to feed the brain cells. Up to 75 percent of the brain's

I have all the energy I need when I wake up in the morning and don't feel compelled to eat until I'm hungry around noon or 1 p.m. I maintain muscle mass and have discovered that I function optimally on fewer calories than I thought necessary.

energy requirements can be met by ketones. Of course, that means that glucose still provides 25 percent of the brain's energy requirements. So does this mean that we have to eat for our brains to function?

Not really. Between the glucose we have already stored away in the form of body fat and what the liver produces in gluconeogenesis, we have plenty of fuel when no food is available. Even prolonged fasting won't send blood glucose levels dangerously low.

Myth #4: Fasting Results in Overeating

Does fasting provoke compensatory overeating? Many authorities warn against missing even a single meal because it could make you extra hungry and unable to avoid temptations, leading to overeating and ultimately no weight loss.

Studies of caloric intake do, in fact, show a slight increase on the first day after fasting. On the day after a one-day fast, average caloric intake increases from 2,436 to 2,914. But if you factor in what would have normally been consumed during that two-day period, 4,872 calories, there is still a net deficit of 1,958 calories. The increased calories don't come close to making up for the lack of calories on the fasting day.

Interestingly, with repeated fasting, you may see the opposite effect. In the Intensive Dietary Management clinic, my personal experience with hundreds of fasting patients shows that, over time, appetite tends to decrease as the fasting duration increases.

Myth #5: Fasting Deprives the Body of Nutrients

There are two main types of nutrients, micronutrients and macronutrients. Micronutrients are vitamin and minerals that are provided by the diet and are required for overall health. Macronutrients are proteins, fats, and carbohydrates.

Micronutrient deficiency is rare in the developed world. With shorter fasting periods (less than twenty-four hours), there is ample opportunity before and after the fast to eat nutrient-dense foods to make up for missed meals. For longer fasts, it is a good idea to take a general multivitamin. The longest fast recorded lasted 382 days, and a simple multivitamin prevented any vitamin deficiencies.

Of the three major macronutrients, there are no essential carbohydrates that the body needs to function, so it is impossible to become carbohydrate deficient. However, there are certain proteins and fats that we have to get in our diet. These are called the essential amino acids (the building blocks of proteins) and essential fatty acids. These cannot be manufactured by the body and must be obtained in the diet.

The body normally loses both essential amino acids and essential fatty acids in urine and stool. During fasting, it reduces these losses to hang onto much of the necessary nutrients. Bowel movements usually decrease during fasting—since no food is going into the stomach, there is less stool formation—and this helps to prevent loss of protein in the stool. Essential nutrients, particularly nitrogen, can be lost through the urine. Nitrogen in the urine is a sign of protein metabolism, and as protein metabolism decreases during fasting, nitrogen in the urine decreases significantly, to almost negligible levels. To further preserve proteins, the body breaks old proteins down into their component amino acids and recycles these into new proteins. By keeping essential nutrients in the body instead of excreting them, the body is able to recycle many of them during fasting.

Of course, no matter how good the body is at compensating, fasting means we're not consuming essential fatty acids and amino acids. Before and after fasting, it can be helpful to follow a low-carbohydrate diet, which increases the percentage of fats and proteins consumed, so the body has more stored up for a rainy day.

Children, pregnant women, and breastfeeding women have a greater need for nutrients than others. In these situations, recycling old proteins and fats isn't enough—new ones are needed to grow and build tissue. For these people, fasting is not a good option. (See Chapter 10 for more on who should not fast.)

Myth #6: "It's Just Crazy"

This always seems to be the fallback position of those who can't think of any other reason why fasting should not be attempted. The science is clear. Obesity, at its very core, involves some form of overeating. This is true whether you believe it is caused by consuming too many calories, carbohydrates, or fats. Fasting helps in all these cases. Its effectiveness is unquestioned. After all, if you don't eat anything at all, don't you think you would lose weight?

The only two remaining questions are:

- *Is it healthy?* The answer to this is *yes*. We'll talk more about why in upcoming chapters.

- *Can you do it?* Absolutely. Millions of people worldwide have fasted for weight loss (and many other reasons). This book is here to help you get started.

References

A. M. Johnstone, P. Faber, E. R. Gibney, M. Elia, G. Horgan, B. E. Golden, and R. J. Stubbs, "Effect of an Acute Fast on Energy Compensation and Feeding Behaviour in Lean Men and Women," *International Journal of Obesity* 26, no. 12 (2002): 1623–8.

Ancel Keys, Josef Brožek, Austin Henschel, Olaf Mickelsen, and Henry Longstreet Taylor, *The Biology of Human Starvation*, 2 vols. (Minneapolis, MN: University of Minnesota Press, 1950).

Christian Zauner, Bruno Schneeweiss, Alexander Kranz, Christian Madl, Klaus Ratheiser, Ludwig Kramer, Erich Roth, Barbara Schneider, and Kurt Lenz, "Resting Energy Expenditure in Short-Term Starvation Is Increased as a Result of an Increase in Serum Norepinephrine," *American Journal of Clinical Nutrition* 71, no. 6 (2000): 1511–5.

E. O. Diaz, A. M. Prentice, G. R. Goldberg, P. R. Murgatroyd, and W. A. Coward, "Metabolic Response to Experimental Overfeeding in Lean and Overweight Healthy Volunteers," *American Journal of Clinical Nutrition* 56, no. 4 (1992): 641–55.

Helene Nørrelund, K. Sreekumaran Nair, Jens Otto Lunde Jørgensen, Jens Sandahl Christiansen, and Niels Møller, "The Protein-Retaining Effects of Growth Hormone During Fasting Involve Inhibition of Muscle-Protein Breakdown," *Diabetes* 50, no. 1 (2001): 96–104.

Leonie K. Heilbronn, Steven R. Smith, Corby K. Martin, Stephen D. Anton, and Eric Ravussin, "Alternate-Day Fasting in Nonobese Subjects: Effects on Body Weight, Body Composition, and Energy Metabolism," *American Journal of Clinical Nutrition* 81, no. 1 (2005): 69–73.

Marshall D. McCue, ed., *Comparative Physiology of Fasting, Starvation, and Food Limitation* (New York: Springer-Verlag Berlin Heidelberg, 2012).

Surabhi Bhutani, Monica C. Klempel, Reed A. Berger, and Krista A. Varady, "Improvements in Coronary Heart Disease Risk Indicators by Alternate-Day Fasting Involve Adipose Tissue Modulations," *Obesity* 18, no. 11 (2010): 2152–9.

Chapter 4
THE ADVANTAGES OF FASTING

Fasting's most obvious benefit is weight loss. However, there are a myriad of benefits beyond this, many of which were widely known before the modern era. It was once common for people to fast for a certain period of time for health benefits. These fasting periods were often called "cleanses," "detoxifications," or "purifications," and people believed that they would clear their bodies of toxins and rejuvenate themselves. They were more correct than they knew. Fasting:

Improves mental clarity and concentration

Induces weight and body fat loss

Lowers blood sugar levels

Improves insulin sensitivity

Increases energy

Improves fat-burning

Lowers blood cholesterol

Prevents Alzheimer's disease

Extends life

Reverses the aging process

Decreases inflammation

We'll talk more about these health benefits in later chapters. But why is fasting better than other diets? We'll look at the advantages to fasting in this chapter.

Diets Fail

One main problem of the diets that have the health benefits listed above is that these are often very difficult to follow, as I discovered when working with my patients with obesity and type 2 diabetes.

Obesity and type 2 diabetes are both problems of excessive insulin. Since refined carbohydrates are a prime contributor to high insulin levels, the natural place to start with my patients was a low-carbohydrate diet. Protein, especially animal proteins (dairy and meat), can also stimulate insulin production, and excessive intake of these foods can slow down progress. And processed foods also play a key role in disease. So, the best diet would emphasize whole, unprocessed foods. It would be low in refined carbohydrates and high in natural fats with a moderate amount of protein.

Multiple peer-reviewed studies have shown that this kind of diet has excellent results for type 2 diabetes and is very safe. So that's what I started with in working with my patients at the Intensive Dietary Management Program. I counseled them on reducing sugars and refined carbohydrates and replacing them with natural, unprocessed foods. I gave lectures. I followed up. I begged. I cajoled. I reviewed page after page of food diaries. *And it just did not work.*

The diet could be successful, but only if it was properly followed, and it was simply too complicated for many of my patients. They would return food diaries filled with noodles and bread and still claim they were following a low-carbohydrate diet. Pitas, naan, and other flatbreads somehow were not considered "bread." They simply did not understand what was being asked of them. These were not, after all, people obsessed with nutrition who spent every spare minute reading medical journals. They had full-time jobs and families to take care of, and trying to break their dietary habits of the last fifty years proved to be very challenging. Also, because this diet was almost the opposite of conventional dietary advice, it was often hard for people to accept that it was actually good for them.

But I couldn't just give up. Their health and, indeed, their very lives depended upon the proper treatment. Type 2 diabetes is a terrible disease. It is by far the leading cause of blindness, amputation, and kidney failure in North America. Diabetes is also a leading contributor to heart attacks, stroke, and other cardiovascular diseases. Type 2 diabetes is a dietary disease, and it requires a dietary solution. Most importantly, it is a *curable* disease.

What I needed was a new strategy. The overall goal was not necessarily to reduce carbohydrate intake. The goal was to reduce insulin levels, and cutting carbohydrates was only one method of achieving that goal. Yet all foods, to varying degrees, stimulate the release of insulin. So the most efficient method of lowering insulin would be to eat nothing at all. In other words: to fast.

I didn't need to reinvent the wheel. People are always drawn to the latest and greatest diet trend, the next superfood, like quinoa, acai berries, or kale chips. But what are the chances that, after thousands of years of human history, we will find the "next great thing" now? The thing that we can't live without, despite having lived without it for thousands of years?

Fasting is the oldest dietary intervention in the world. It is profoundly different from all other dietary strategies. It is not the latest and greatest but the tried and true. It is not something to do but something to *not* do. Because it differs from conventional dieting in many important ways, fasting carries many distinct advantages.

Advantage #1: It's Simple

Because there is no consensus as to what constitutes a healthy diet, my patients were often confused. Should they go low-fat? Low-carb? Low-calorie? Low-sugar? Low glycemic index?

Fasting, by taking a completely different approach, is much easier to understand. It is so simple that it can be explained in two sentences: Eat nothing. Drink water, tea, coffee, or bone broth. That's it.

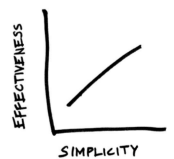

This work is a derivative of "Effective Simplicity" by www.behaviorgap.com, used under CC BY.

I initially become interested in fasting for its applications in healing the gut. Many of the patients I work with have severe food sensitivities even though they have very healthy diets. For these patients there is usually some underlying inflammatory or infectious issue. Fasting can provide instantaneous relief of symptoms and aids in supporting recovery from the underlying issue.

Diets can fail because they are ineffective. But they just as surely fail if people are not able to follow them. The most obvious benefit to fasting is that its simplicity makes it effective. When it comes to dietary rules, the simpler, the better.

Advantage #2: It's Free

I prefer patients to eat organic, local grass-fed beef and organic vegetables, and avoid white bread and other highly processed foods. However, the truth is that these kinds of healthy foods are often very expensive; they can cost ten times as much as processed foods.

Grains enjoy substantial government subsidies, making them far cheaper than other foods. This means that a pound of fresh cherries may cost $6.99, while an entire loaf of bread will cost $1.99. An entire box of pasta may cost only $0.99 on sale. Feeding a family on a budget is a lot easier when you buy pasta and white bread.

If a diet is unaffordable, it does not truly matter if it is effective. The price makes it ineffective for those who cannot afford to follow it. This should not doom them to a lifetime of type 2 diabetes and disability.

Fasting is free. In fact, not only is it free, it actually saves money because you do not need to buy any food at all! There are no expensive foods. There are no expensive supplements. There are no meal replacement bars, shakes, or medications. The price of fasting is zero.

Advantage #3: It's Convenient

It is healthy to always eat a home-cooked, prepared-from-scratch meal. However, many people, myself included, simply do not have the time or inclination to cook. Between work, school, family, kids, after-school activities, and after-work activities, there just is not a lot of time left over. Cooking involves preparation time, shopping time, cooking time, and cleanup time. Everything takes time, and time seems to be one commodity that's in constant shortage.

The number of meals eaten away from home has been steadily increasing over the past few decades. While many try to support the "slow food" movement, it is clear that they are fighting a losing battle against fast food.

Meals Eaten at Home vs Away from Home

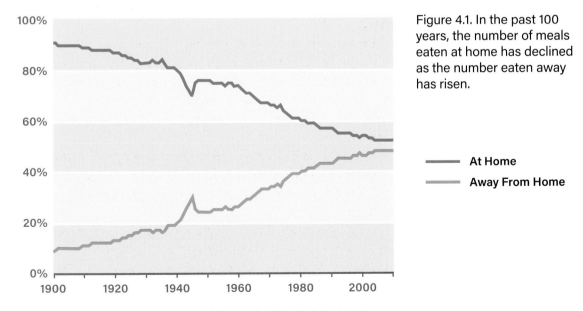

Figure 4.1. In the past 100 years, the number of meals eaten at home has declined as the number eaten away has risen.

Source: Derek Thompson, "Cheap Eats: How America Spends Money on Food," *The Atlantic,* March 8, 2013.

So asking people to devote themselves to home cooking, as well-intentioned as it may be, is not going to be a winning strategy. Fasting, on the other hand, is the exact opposite. There is no time spent buying groceries, preparing ingredients, cooking, and cleaning up. It is a way to simplify your life.

There is nothing easier than fasting, because fasting involves doing nothing. Most diets tell you what to do. Fasting tells you not to do anything. It doesn't get easier than that.

Advantage #4: You Can Enjoy Life's Little Pleasures

Some diets advise people to never, ever again eat ice cream or desserts. Good advice for weight loss, obviously. But I don't think it is actually very practical advice. Sure, you might be able to swear off desserts for six months or a year, but for life? And would you really want to? Think about it. Imagine the joy of savoring the cake and champagne at your best friend's wedding. Do we need to deny ourselves that little bit of pleasure forever? Enjoy a birthday salad instead of birthday cake? Thanksgiving kale chips! All-you-can-eat Brussels sprouts! Yes, life just got a little less sparkly. Forever is a long time.

Now, I am not saying that you should eat dessert every single day. However, fasting restores the ability to occasionally enjoy that dessert by balancing out the feast. It is, after all, the cycle of life. Feasts follow fasts. Fasts follow feasts. This is how we have always lived. Birthdays, weddings, holidays, and other special occasions have always, throughout human history, been celebrated with feasts. But those feasts should be followed by fasts.

If you have a wedding coming up, you are more than entitled to look forward to enjoying yourself and eating decadent, delicious wedding cake. And when you fast regularly, you do not need to feel guilty about enjoying one of life's little pleasures, because you can make up for it.

The most important aspect of fasting is fitting it into your life. There will be times where it is not appropriate to fast. Who wants to forever be the party pooper who won't eat this and won't drink that? You can indulge yourself, as long you balance that with some abstinence. Fasting is really about *balance*. It is the flip side, the

B-side, of eating. Balance the time that you are eating and the time you are not eating to remain healthy. When those two fall out of balance, that's when we get into trouble.

Advantage #5: It's Powerful

Many type 2 diabetics are morbidly obese and highly insulin-resistant. Occasionally, even a strict ketogenic diet (one that's very low in carbohydrate, moderate in protein, and high in fat) is not strong enough to reverse their disease. The quickest and most efficient way to lower insulin and insulin resistance is fasting. It has unrivaled power to break through weight-loss plateaus and reduce the need for insulin.

From a therapeutic standpoint, a key advantage of fasting is that it has no upper limit—there's no maximum amount of time that you can fast. The world record for fasting was 382 days, during which the patient suffered no ill effects. So if fasting occasionally isn't working, all you need to do is increase the frequency or length of time you fast, until you reach your goal.

Compare this to medications. Virtually every drug has a maximum dose. If you take penicillin for an infection, for example, there is a maximum dose above which there is little extra benefit and the medication may become toxic. At that point, if you still have the infection, you need to change medications. The same applies to low-carbohydrate or low-fat diets. Once you hit zero carbs or fat, you can go no further with that diet. There is a maximum dose. Once you reach the maximum, you need to change diets to gain any extra effect.

FASTING ALL-STARS DR. BERT HERRING

The summary benefits of a successful fasting schedule maintained over a month or more include appetite correction, loss of surplus fat, decreased inflammation (measured in symptom severity or C-reactive protein, CRP), decreased blood sugars in diabetics (measured by blood glucose or HbA1c), and decreased blood pressure in hypertensive people.

FASTING—
UNLIMITED POWER

Fasting has no ceiling, which offers significant therapeutic flexibility. In other words, you can keep fasting until the desired effects are seen. The dose can go up indefinitely. Ask yourself this question: if you don't eat, will you lose weight? Of course. Even a child understands that you *must* lose weight. So fasting's efficacy is unquestioned. It is the most powerful method of weight loss available. It is only a question of safety and compliance. For more complicated or serious cases of obesity, we can simply increase the dose.

What's more, low-fat diets, low-carbohydrate diets, Paleo diets, and indeed almost all diets work for some people but not others, and when a diet doesn't work for you, there is little you can do to make it more effective. However, with fasting, all you need to do is increase the amount of time spent fasting. The longer you go, the more likely you are to lose weight—and it will happen eventually.

Advantage #6: It's Flexible

Some diet plans advocate eating as soon as you wake up and then every two and a half hours during the day. Some people have had good results with such a diet. However, finding or packing something to eat six or seven or eight times a day is very intrusive. I could not imagine interrupting my life every two and a half hours to snack. It's too disruptive on an already hectic schedule. And it's simply not necessary.

Fasting can be done at any time. There is no set duration. You may fast for sixteen hours or sixteen days. You can mix and match time periods. You are never locked into a pattern. You may fast for one day this week, five days the next, and two days the week after. Life is unpredictable. Fasting fits wherever you need it to.

Fasting can be done anywhere. It does not matter if you live in the United States, the United Kingdom, or the United Arab Emirates. You may live in the polar desert of the Arctic or the sandy desert of Saudi Arabia. It matters not at all. Once again, because fasting is about *not* doing something, it simplifies our life. It adds simplicity where other diets add complexity.

If you do not feel well for any reason, you simply stop fasting. It is entirely reversible within minutes. If you wish to stop fasting for several weeks for personal or medical reasons, then you may do so. If you want to indulge during the Christmas holidays or during a summer cruise, you can do that as well. Simply get back on the program once you are finished.

Compare this to bariatric surgery (sometimes called "stomach stapling"). It has helped many people lose a lot of weight, at least in the short term. But this surgery has tons of complications, almost all of which are irreversible. And you cannot simply reverse the surgery itself. It's permanent. If you are doing poorly, that's simply too bad. Fasting, on the other hand, is completely within your control; you may fast or stop fasting anytime you wish.

Advantage #7: It Works with Any Diet

Here is the biggest advantage of all: fasting can be added to any diet. That is because fasting is not about something you do; it's about something you do *not* do. It is subtraction rather than addition. This makes fasting fundamentally different from almost every diet imaginable.

You don't eat meat? You can still fast.

You don't eat wheat? You can still fast.

You have a nut allergy? You can still fast.

You don't have time? You can still fast.

You don't have money? You can still fast.

You are traveling all the time? You can still fast.

You don't cook? You can still fast.

You are eighty years old? You can still fast.

You have problems chewing? You can still fast.

What could possibly be simpler?

Fasting can be flexible. The day of a fast can be moved around and doesn't have to be set in stone. If I've got a particularly important meeting on a Thursday, for example—and feel it would be best to eat a breakfast—I can either change the hours I fast or just move it to another day in the week.

—**Stella B., Leeds, UK**

ELIZABETH

FASTING SUCCESS STORY

I grew up in South Africa and was overweight most of my life, with periods of weight loss due to yo-yo dieting. In 2002 I went on a fat-free, high-carbohydrate diet for two years. Early in 2004 I was diagnosed with type 2 diabetes, high cholesterol, and high blood pressure, and started on medication. My father and siblings were also on medication for these concerns.

At 105 kg (231 pounds), I switched from my fat-free, high-carbohydrate diet to a low-carbohydrate, severely calorie-restricted diet. My weight went down to 75 kg (165 pounds) over about eighteen months, but the diet was so restrictive it was not sustainable. Inevitably, my weight climbed back up. At the end of 2010, I was horrified when an ultrasound showed that I had nonalcoholic fatty liver disease.

In April 2011, my doctor added insulin injections to my type 2 diabetes medications. He said I had to increase the insulin dose until my blood glucose level was down, with no other explanation— so I did just that! Late in 2011 I was injecting 120 units of long-acting insulin every night and 80 units of rapid-acting insulin with each meal. I was also still taking my other diabetes medication morning and night.

After I started taking insulin, no matter what I did or how hard I exercised, I could not lose weight—even when I quit carbohydrates. I knew it had something to do with the insulin. Fast-forward to January 2015: I had had enough. I began cutting carbohydrates again and started a thirty-minute high-intensity interval training class. My glucose levels were dropping to about 2.3 mmol/L. Then I came across an article by Dr. Fung, who had just presented at the Low Carb High Fat Convention in Cape Town, saying type 2 diabetes could be reversed. I watched his YouTube presentations, and for the first time, I found something that made sense. I immediately decided that quitting insulin was my first priority, but I could not find a single dietitian or doctor in South Africa who would help me.

JANUARY 2015

Weight	96 kg (212 pounds)
Fasting glucose	9.5 mmol/L
HbA1c	7.6%
Insulin dosage	360 units/day

So I read more on Dr. Fung's Intensive Dietary Management blog, and toward the end of

February I started a fasting regimen along with low-carbohydrate meals. I cut all my insulin doses in half. I began with three days of fasting a week. On fasting days, I drank coffee with cream in the morning and water with a slice of lemon in it the remainder of the day. Later, I learned that you don't really need breakfast, so I started eating just one meal in the late afternoon on nonfasting days.

My glucose levels continued to drop, so I quit all injected insulin and continued to eat a low-carb, Paleo-style diet (in other words, *real food*). My weight was slowly coming down and the needle on the scale was 87.8 kg (194 pounds). I had lost a total of 6.2 kg (14 pounds) of body fat (2.9% of my total), and my waistline dropped 35 cm (14 inches).

JUNE 2015

Weight	79.7 kg (176 pounds)
Fasting glucose	7.6 mmol/L
HbA1c	6.2%
Insulin dosage	none

By the beginning of June, my weight was 79.7 kg (176 pounds) and I had lost a total of 13.03 kg (29 pounds) of body fat (7.3%) and a total of 46.5 cm (18 inches) from my waist.

I continued my fasting regimen, and in August I finally found a physician to help me the last bit of the way. My results have astounded various people in various ways, including some friends in the medical profession who were too polite to tell me that they thought I was nuts!

NOVEMBER 2015

Weight	68 kg (150 pounds)
Fasting glucose	5.9 mmol/L
HbA1c	5.3%
Insulin dosage	none

It's the end of November 2015, and I now weigh 68 kg (150 pounds) and have lost a total of 20.64 kg (46 pounds) of body fat (12.4%) and a total of 77.5 cm (31 inches) from my waist.

I realize that I am always going to struggle with my love of carbohydrates, especially bread and fruit, but I know that my way of eating—real foods combined with a fasting regimen—is sustainable. As Dr. Fung put it, there are times of feast, but it is easy enough to balance these with times of famine (fasting). I feel so much better having lost so much weight, and I have lots of energy when fasting.

Chapter 5
FASTING FOR WEIGHT LOSS

Long-term dieting is an exercise in futility. All diets—whether the Mediterranean diet, the Atkins diet, or even the old-fashioned low-fat, low-calorie diet—seem to produce weight loss in the short term. But after some initial success, weight loss plateaus, and the dreaded weight regain follows. Even low-carbohydrate diets, which are proven to result in more weight loss than other diets in the short term, show the same inexorable plateau and weight regain. This relentless regain occurs despite continued dietary compliance and regardless of dietary strategy.

In other words, eventually, all diets fail. The question is, *why?*

"Eat Less, Move More" Doesn't Work

Have you ever heard the phrase "The proof is in the pudding"? The original version was actually "The proof of the pudding is in the eating." It means that to really judge whether something is successful or not, you must look at the end results. Just because you *think* something will work does not necessarily mean it will.

So let's apply this to obesity. The dominant nutritional paradigm of the last half century has been "calories in, calories out." The idea is that consuming fewer calories than are used will ultimately lead to lasting weight loss. Dietary fat, being calorically dense (there are nine calories in every gram of fat, compared to four in every gram of carbohydrate or protein), was believed to be especially fattening.

The commonly recommended weight-loss approach of a low-fat, low-calorie diet combined with increased exercise—all aimed at increasing the number of calories burned while reducing the number of calories consumed—can be neatly summarized as "eat less, move more." There is certainly a logic at work here, and we can imagine all kinds of reasons why it *should* work, but does it? What are the results of this approach?

As you and I both know, this dietary approach has been widely advocated over the past few decades and has created a huge, rampant global obesity epidemic. The Centers for Disease Control and Prevention in Atlanta closely tracks obesity trends in the United States, and according to its data, in 2015, no state had an obesity rate *below* 20 percent. Only twenty years earlier, in 1995, no state had an obesity rate *above* 20 percent.

So we have two incontrovertible facts:

Fact #1—Over the past twenty years, conventional weight-loss advice has called for eating less and moving more.

Fact #2—Over the past twenty years, obesity rates have exploded.

Considering these facts together, there are only two possible conclusions. The first is that our standard dietary advice is good, but people are simply not following it. This would be a real stretch of the imagination. When it comes to health, people really do listen to their doctors, as we can see when we look at other lifestyle changes doctors began to recommend. When doctors advised people to stop smoking, they stopped smoking. In the mid-1960s, as the data linking lung cancer and smoking became clear, the Surgeon General of the United States first issued a public health warning. Cigarette consumption shortly thereafter began its relentless downward trend, which was accelerated by the Surgeon General's report on secondhand smoke.

When doctors advised people to watch their blood pressure and cholesterol, they watched their blood pressure and cholesterol. Yet somehow, when doctors advised people to eat less and move more, they didn't? Doubtful.

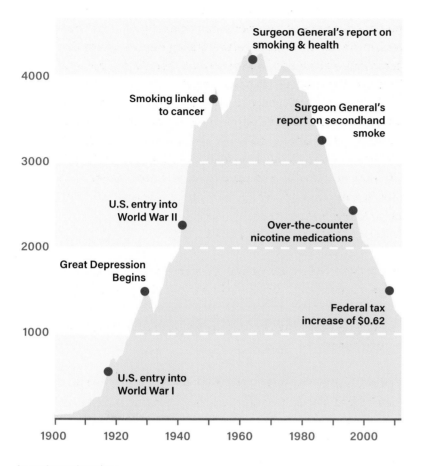

Historic Cigarette Consumption

Surgeon General's report on smoking & health

Smoking linked to cancer

Surgeon General's report on secondhand smoke

U.S. entry into World War II

Over-the-counter nicotine medications

Great Depression Begins

Federal tax increase of $0.62

U.S. entry into World War I

4000
3000
2000
1000

1900   1920   1940   1960   1980   2000

Figure 5.1. Adult per capita cigarette consumption, 1900–2012. When doctors started telling people that smoking was bad for their health, people listened and smoking rates declined.

Source: SurgeonGeneral.gov

This way of thinking is also known as "blaming the victim." We assume the advice is good and therefore, if it fails, it must be because the person didn't really follow the advice. This shifts the blame from the advice-giver to the advice-taker.

Americans have, in fact, followed the government's nutritional guidelines. The USDA's first *Dietary Guidelines for Americans* was released in 1977. It recommended that Americans adjust their diets to meet two specific goals: increase consumption of carbohydrates and reduce intake of total fat. Although caloric reduction was not a specified goal, the reduction in dietary fat was expected to reduce calories, since fat is calorically dense compared to carbohydrates.

Since 1970, consumption of vegetables, fruits, and grains has increased, and consumption of red meat, eggs, and animal fats has declined, just as the USDA's dietary guidelines recommended. But the promised benefits never materialized.

The second possible conclusion—the only one that remains—is that *the advice to eat less and move more is simply wrong.* And scientific studies back this up.

We've known about the abysmal success rate of the caloric-reduction approach—the one that's based on simply reducing calories consumed and increasing calories burned—for decades.

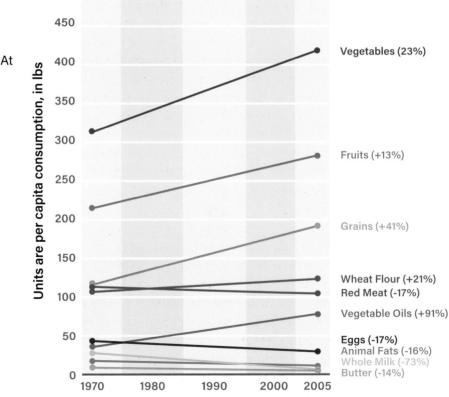

Figure 5.2. Since 1970, Americans have largely followed the government's dietary recommendations. At the same time, the obesity epidemic has exploded.

Source: Wells and Buzby, "Dietary Assessment of Major Trends in U.S. Food Consumption, 1970–2005."

A 1959 study estimated its failure rate at a sky-high 98 percent. Only 2 percent of dieters using a caloric-reduction strategy were able to maintain a twenty-pound weight loss for two years.

More recently, in 2015, researchers in the United Kingdom reviewed the weight-loss rates of more than 175,000 obese men and women over the previous nine years. The probability of achieving a normal weight by caloric reduction alone was 0.8 percent in women and 0.47 percent in men. So the best-case scenario using conventional calorie-counting methods is a 99.2 percent failure rate.

Even the very best study ever done on caloric reduction as a path to lasting weight loss showed that it failed. The Women's Health Initiative, a gigantic randomized controlled trial, followed almost fifty thousand women over seven and a half years. One group of the women followed a low-fat, low-calorie diet high in grains, fruits, and vegetables and reduced their total daily calories by 361 calories; their percentage of calories from fat was reduced from 38.8 percent to 29.8 percent. They also increased their amount of exercise by 14 percent. The other group followed their usual diet. The expected weight loss for the low-calorie, increased-exercise group was thirty-six pounds per year, or 252 pounds over seven years. The other group was not expected to see any weight loss.

The final results were a complete shock to everybody involved. The actual difference in weight loss between the two groups was not even two pounds! Worse still, the average waist size in the low-calorie, increased-exercise group grew from 35 to 35.4 inches. These women who so carefully followed the "eat less, move more" strategy for so long actually ended up fatter than ever.

There's a better-known example to be found in *The Biggest Loser*, a long-running reality TV show that pits obese contestants against one another in a bid to lose the most weight. While short-term results are often stunning, contestants nearly always regain weight after filming ends. Kai Hibbard, the winner of season three, said of participating on the show, "It was the biggest mistake of my life." Season two's Suzanne Mendonca says that there is never a reunion show because "we're all fat again."

Women's Health Initiative: Eat Less, Move More

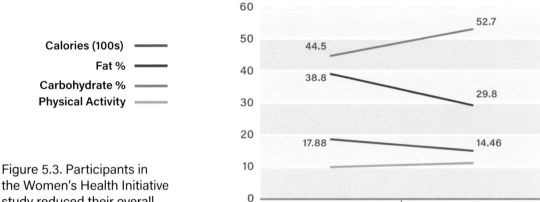

Calories (100s) ━━━
Fat % ━━━
Carbohydrate % ━━━
Physical Activity ━━━

Figure 5.3. Participants in the Women's Health Initiative study reduced their overall calories and fat consumption while increasing their exercise and carbohydrate consumption over seven years.

Source: Data from Howard et al., "Low-Fat Dietary Pattern and Weight Change over 7 Years: The Women's Health Initiative Dietary Modification Trial."

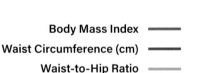
Body Mass Index ━━━
Waist Circumference (cm) ━━━
Waist-to-Hip Ratio ━━━

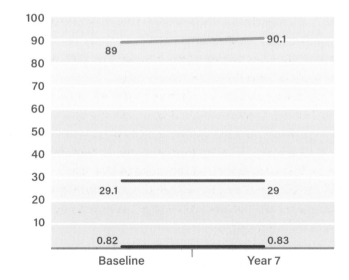

Figure 5.4. Despite a low-fat, low-calorie diet (see Figure 5.3), participants in the Women's Health Initiative saw little change in their BMI or waist-to-hip ratio, and their waist circumference actually increased slightly.

Source: Data from Howard et al., "Low-Fat Dietary Pattern and Weight Change over 7 Years: The Women's Health Initiative Dietary Modification Trial."

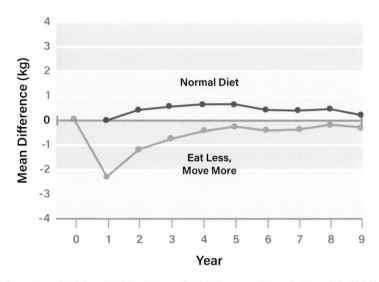

Figure 5.5. Over nine years, women adhering to a calorie-restricted diet showed no weight-loss benefits over those eating a normal diet.

Source: Howard et al., "Low-Fat Dietary Pattern and Weight Change over 7 Years: The Women's Health Initiative Dietary Modification Trial."

But why should this happen? The *Biggest Loser* diet restricts calories to 70 percent of baseline energy requirements, which usually means 1200 to 1500 calories per day. This is combined with vigorous physical exertion for several hours per day, six days a week. This is the classic "eat less, move more" advice given by dietitians and health-care professionals everywhere. No wonder the *Biggest Loser* diet ranked number three in weight-loss diets according to *US News & World Report* in 2015.

A study of *Biggest Loser* contestants showed that in thirty weeks of filming, average weight dropped from 329 pounds to 202 pounds. That's an average decrease of 127 pounds! Body fat dropped, on average, from 49 percent to 28 percent. Almost all of the weight lost was fat mass, as opposed to lean tissue, or "fat-free mass". (There is inevitably some lean tissue lost along with fat, but this is generally skin and connective tissue, not necessarily muscle.) Wow! Amazing!

Unfortunately, those results simply didn't last.

Six years after their almost miraculous weight loss, thirteen of the fourteen contestants studied had regained the weight they'd lost. This is a failure rate of 93 percent. The main reason for the weight regain is that the contestants' metabolisms had slowed significantly (we'll explain why later in this chapter). Danny Cahill, the winner of Season 8, lost 239 pounds during the competition. However, his body was now burning 800 calories less per day than it had previously. This proved to be an insurmountable obstacle to lasting weight loss, and sure enough, he, along with almost all the other contestants, ended up regaining all their hard-lost weight.

But I probably didn't really need to convince you that "eat less, move more" doesn't work. You already knew that. For the vast majority of people, personal experience confirms this epic fail. Yes, studies prove that it does not work, but just as significantly, so do the bitter experiences of the millions of people who have tried it. Ninety-nine percent failure rate? Sounds about right to me.

This is the cruel hoax of the "eat less, move more" strategy. It is cruel because all of our trusted health sources tell us it should work, and when it fails, we blame ourselves.

Here's the thing, though. Let's say, for the sake of argument, that when followed to the letter, "eat less, move more" does work.

Biggest Loser Contestants Lost Weight During the Show

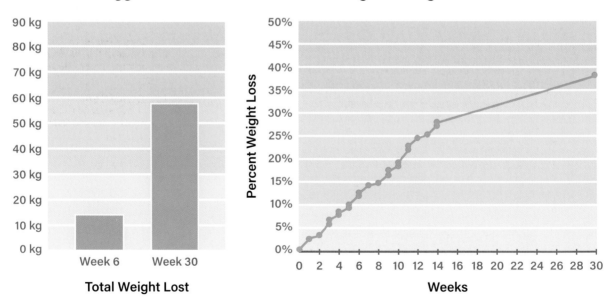

Figure 5.6. During thirty weeks of filming, *Biggest Loser* contestants showed amazing weight-loss results.

Source: Johannsen et al., "Metabolic Slowing with Massive Weight Loss Despite Preservation of Fat-Free Mass."

In the end, it actually doesn't matter. Whether it's good advice that people don't follow or bad advice that people do follow, the result is the same: it doesn't produce weight loss. And if the end results are bad—and they are!—then the advice is bad. The proof is in the pudding.

What is to be done? The only logical conclusion is to change that advice. We need a new strategy—fasting.

Biggest Loser Contestants Regained Weight After the Show

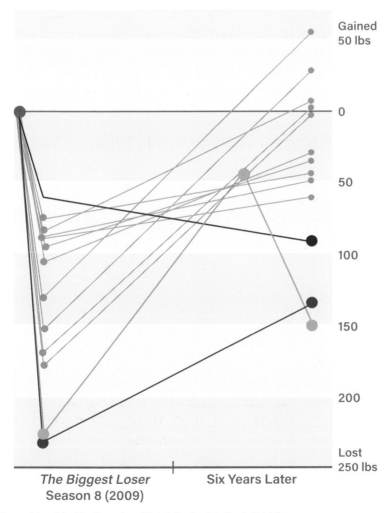

Gained 50 lbs

0

50

100

150

200

Lost 250 lbs

The Biggest Loser Season 8 (2009)

Six Years Later

Figure 5.7. After six years, nearly all the *Biggest Loser* contestants had regained the weight they lost.

—— **Erinn Egbert** is the only contestant who has not regained weight since the show.

—— **Rudy Pauls** regained most of the weight he'd lost before having bariatric surgery.

—— **Danny Cahill** lost the most weight to win the competition, but he's put back on over 100 pounds.

Source: Kolata, "After 'The Biggest Loser,' Their Bodies Fought to Regain Weight"

Biggest Loser Contestants Have Slowed Metabolisms

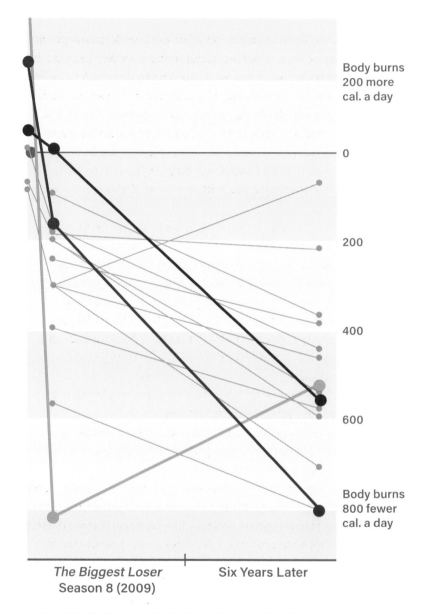

Figure 5.8. Slowing metabolisms made it impossible for most *Biggest Loser* contestants to maintain their weight loss.

—— Erinn Egbert
is the only contestant who has not regained weight since the show.

—— Rudy Pauls
regained most of the weight he'd lost before having bariatric surgery.

—— Danny Cahill
now burns 600 fewer calories a day than he did during the show.

Body burns 200 more cal. a day

0

200

400

600

Body burns 800 fewer cal. a day

The Biggest Loser
Season 8 (2009)

Six Years Later

Source: Kolata, "After 'The Biggest Loser,' Their Bodies Fought to Regain Weight."

Why "Eat Less, Move More" Fails:
How Our Bodies Really Use Calories

The reason "eat less, move more" doesn't work for weight loss is that it's based on a false idea about how our bodies use calories: the single-compartment model. According to this model, the body reduces all foods to simple calories and stores those calories for use in what we can think of as a single compartment; then, the body accesses that compartment to use the calories for exercise and basal metabolism (remember, that refers to the body's basic functions, such as breathing, removing toxins from the bloodstream, digesting foods, and so on—all these require energy from calories).

This model is like a bathroom sink. Calories, like water, can flow into or out of this sink. Excess calories are held in this sink and can be easily accessed if our bodies require more calories—for example, exercise would drain calories out of this sink. There is no distinction made between any of the storage forms of calories. Whether calories are stored as glucose, which is used for immediate energy; glycogen, which is used in the intermediate time frame; or fat, which is long-term energy storage, all calories are treated equally.

However, this model is known to be a complete fabrication. It does not exist except in our imaginations.

It is more accurate to use a two-compartment model, because there are two distinct ways energy is stored in the body: as glycogen in the liver and as body fat.

When we eat, our body derives energy from three main sources: glucose (carbohydrates), fat, and protein. Only two of these are stored for later use, glucose and fat—the body can't store protein, so excess protein that can't be used right away is converted to glucose. Glucose is stored in the liver as glycogen, but the liver's capacity for storing glycogen is limited. Once glycogen stores are full, excess calories must be stored as body fat. Dietary fat is absorbed directly into the bloodstream without passing through the liver, and what's not used is stored as body fat. This was one of the reasons why low-fat diets were initially recommended, but the immediate destination of ingested calories is not the main determinant of weight gain.

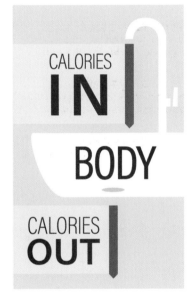

The single-compartment model of calorie storage and use.

Think of glycogen as a refrigerator. It's designed for short-term storage of food; it's very easy to move food in and out, but the storage space is limited. Body fat, on the other hand, is more like a basement freezer. It's designed for long-term storage and is more difficult to access, but it has much greater capacity. Plus, you can always add more freezers to the basement if you need them. When we buy groceries, we store food in the refrigerator first, and then when the fridge is full, we store the excess food in the freezer—that is, we store food energy first as glycogen and then, when the space for glycogen is full, as body fat.

Both body fat and glycogen are used for energy in the absence of food, but they aren't used equally or at the same time.

The body prefers to use glycogen for energy rather than body fat. This is logical because it is easier to burn glycogen—in terms of our analogy, it's much easier to get food from the refrigerator in the kitchen than to trek all the way down to the freezer in the basement. And as long as there is food in the fridge, we won't retrieve any from the freezer. In other words, if you need

The two-compartment model of calorie storage and use.

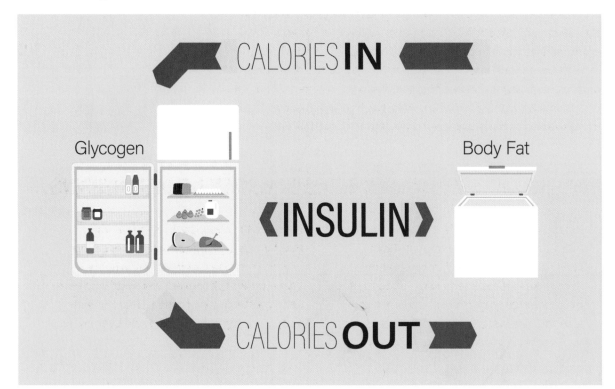

200 calories of energy to go for a walk, the body will get that energy from glycogen as long as it's available—it won't go to the trouble of accessing body fat.

The two compartments, the fridge and the freezer, are not used simultaneously but *sequentially*. You need to (mostly) empty out the fridge before you can use what's in the freezer—you need to burn most of the glycogen before you can burn fat. In essence, the body can burn either sugar or fat, but not both.

Insulin's Crucial Role in Weight Loss and Regain

How easy it is to get to the fat freezer depends upon the hormone insulin. Is the freezer locked away in the basement behind steel gates, or is it located right beside the refrigerator? Insulin levels are the prime determinant.

When we are not eating, insulin levels are low, allowing full access to the fat freezer—the body is able to easily get at the stored fat. With low insulin levels, you don't even have to completely empty the glycogen refrigerator before opening the fat freezer, since it's so easily accessible. Think about your fridge at home. Does it have to be completely empty of everything, including that half-empty bottle of ketchup and tub of yogurt, before you open that pack of burgers from the freezer? Of course not! Similarly, with low insulin levels, the body can burn fat even if there is still some glucose around. That means that if you're

FASTING ALL-STARS | DR. BERT HERRING

After a week or two of fasting for 19 hours a day and eating only within a 5-hour window, I was surprised to see that my excess weight had clearly started to melt away. I had only 20 extra pounds at that time, but the weight bothered me because my efforts to eat less and exercise more had failed to eliminate it. In the years that followed, I kept turning to this eating schedule to lose weight that inevitably accumulated whenever I would drift back to eating 3 meals a day. I found that the wide-interval eating schedule worked every time.

I have done dinner-to-dinner intermittent fasting for a month and a half. I have experienced more energy, and I have been able to increase the amount of weight I'm lifting during my workouts. I average between 2 and 4 pounds per week in weight loss, and I've had a DXA scan that shows the weight I'm losing is fat, not muscle. On top of the weight loss itself, I have lost noticeable inches in my abdominal area. I am also a type 2 diabetic, and intermittent fasting has allowed me to keep my blood sugar levels in a normal range.

—Eric R.,
Ogden, UT

Figure 5.9. From 1922, a girl with type 1 diabetes before and after treatment with insulin.

cutting calories and have low insulin levels, it's easy for your body to compensate for the reduced food energy by getting some fat out of the freezer even if your glycogen fridge isn't completely empty. But the emptier your glycogen fridge, the more likely you will be to use what's in the fat freezer, and the easier it is to get to the freezer, the more likely it is that you will use it.

Not only do low insulin levels *allow* access to the fat freezer, they actually trigger fat-burning for energy. If insulin levels are abnormally low, then fat is continually burned. We see this situation in type 1 diabetes, when the insulin-producing cells in the pancreas are destroyed. As insulin falls to undetectable levels, patients, often children, burn through all their fat stores and are unable to gain weight no matter how many calories they consume. Untreated, this is a fatal disease. Treatment with insulin injections allows them to store fat normally once again.

On the other hand, high insulin levels prevent the body from accessing the fat in the freezer. It is locked away behind steel bars. Insulin inhibits lipolysis—it stops the body from burning fat. High insulin levels, which are normal after meals, signal our body to store some of the incoming energy. Logically, therefore, we also stop burning stored fat (why bother when there's energy from food?).

This doesn't just happen after meals, however—we also see this in diseases of too much insulin. For example, insulin injections, often used in the treatment of diabetes, commonly lead to

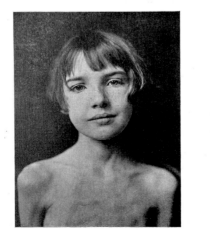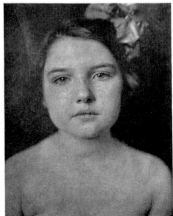

increased fat accumulation because the body is unable to burn fat. (That's great for type 1 diabetics, who have too little fat to begin with, but not so great for type 2 diabetics, who usually have too much.) Insulin resistance, sometimes called prediabetes or metabolic syndrome, is the most common situation where insulin levels are persistently kept abnormally high.

Insulin Resistance

One of insulin's main jobs is to move glucose from the bloodstream into the cells so that it can be used for energy. If you have insulin resistance, your cells are no longer sensitive to insulin. Normal amounts of insulin are not able to move glucose into cells, leading to a buildup of glucose in the blood. To compensate, the body must produce extra insulin to force the glucose in. This leads to constant high insulin levels, which blocks fat-burning. (We'll cover this in more detail in the next chapter, on type 2 diabetes and fasting.)

But what causes insulin resistance in the first place?

The clue lies in its very name. Insulin resistance develops because cells need to resist the effects of too much insulin. The root cause of the problem is consistently high levels of insulin, which creates a vicious cycle: too much insulin creates resistance, insulin resistance triggers higher levels of insulin, and that in turn only serves to stimulate more resistance. The cycle reinforces itself each time it goes around. The way to successfully break the insulin resistance cycle is not to continually increase insulin levels but to drastically *decrease* insulin levels.

This sounds almost counterintuitive, but consider the analogous problem of antibiotic resistance. When an antibiotic is first used, it kills off most bacteria, but a few bacteria are naturally resistant, and these survive—and with the rest of the bacteria gone, they're able to flourish without any competition for resources. These resistant bacteria reproduce and spread, rendering the antibiotic less effective in general—there are fewer bacteria that it will work against. In this case, antibiotics create antibiotic resistance.

How do you stop antibiotic resistance? The knee-jerk reaction is to use even higher doses of antibiotics to kill the resistant bacteria. And this will work for a time, but eventually, the higher dose of antibiotics only creates more resistance. This creates a vicious cycle of antibiotic usage and development of resistance. The answer is the exact opposite: we must severely curtail the use of antibiotics, so resistant bacteria don't flourish.

The same logic applies to insulin resistance. When our cells become less sensitive to insulin, the body's knee-jerk reaction is to increase insulin production. It helps for a while, but over time, this only creates more insulin resistance and triggers the vicious cycle of increasing insulin and increasing resistance. The answer is really the exact opposite: since insulin resistance develops in response to persistently high insulin levels, we must create recurrent periods of *very low* insulin levels.

If we are unable to break the cycle of insulin resistance, then insulin levels remain high. This blocks our ability to burn the body fat we have so carefully stored away. Our body is constantly receiving the signal to store energy as fat and is never told to burn fat. Insulin plays a crucial role in the decision of which fuel to burn.

High Insulin + Reduced Calories = Slowing Metabolism

To find out what all this has to do with losing weight, let's return to the single-compartment and two-compartment models. Remember that the traditional advice to "eat less, move more" for weight loss is based on the single-compartment model, the (incorrect!) idea that all calories are equal and stored in one single compartment, so if you're using more calories than you're consuming, you must be burning body fat. In reality, the body stores energy as both glycogen and body fat—that's the two-compartment model. To burn fat, two things must happen: you must burn through most of your stored glycogen, and insulin levels must drop low enough to release the fat stores.

And neither task is easy. When stored glycogen gets low, your body senses it and starts to get antsy. It triggers hunger signals, so you want to eat more. If you don't eat enough to fill up the glycogen stores but your insulin remains high, body fat can't be released. The body's only remaining option is to decrease your metabolism so that you're burning less energy.

When either food or glycogen is available, we do not use our less-accessible fat stores. This ensures that body fat is only used in times of need. But over decades of abundant glucose, fat stores proliferate because we never allow our fridge to empty. In other words, the food goes into the freezer, but it never gets a chance to come back out. And as insulin resistance progresses, the resulting high insulin levels make it harder and harder to access the fat stores.

The body always wants to stay at a certain weight, and any deviation above or below that weight triggers adaptive mechanisms to get us to return to that weight. That's why, after weight loss, we become hungrier and our metabolism relentlessly slows, so that we have to eat even less just to maintain our lower weight. That's the body trying to get us to gain weight to get us back to our set weight.

The reason the body has to resort to decreasing metabolism and increasing hunger is because insulin remains high, so it doesn't have access to the energy stored as fat. Your body has no other option but to slow metabolism—it's trying to conserve energy because it can't get at the fat freezer. This is why insulin resistance plays such a crucial role in obesity: the high insulin levels tell your body to hang onto body fat and simultaneously trigger the body to lower your metabolism. This inexorably erodes weight-loss efforts. Body weight plateaus and then ruthlessly climbs back up, even as the proper diet is maintained. For some of us, changing what we eat is clearly not enough.

Let's take an example. Suppose you eat 2,000 calories per day. Your weight is stable, so you are burning 2,000 calories per day. There are 3,500 calories in a pound of fat, so if you carry 100 pounds of fat, there are 350,000 calories in fat stores.

Now, let's say you want to lose weight, so you reduce your daily calories to 1,200. Initially, fat will be lost to make up for the reduced calories. However, if you have insulin resistance, then persistently high insulin levels will make it difficult to access fat stores. The high insulin is instructing the body to store energy, not burn it. The body is used to burning 2,000 calories, but now, only 1,200 are available, so it is forced to reduce its energy expenditure to match. Basal metabolic rate decreases to 1,200 calories.

> My insulin resistance made me impervious to lasting weight loss. At age 61, I don't think I had ever gone one day in my life without eating anything, so it was really scary for me to fast. My first fast was for 6 days (about a month ago). I came to realize that hunger pangs are short-lived and pass quickly, making it very doable. I lost 8 pounds that week and have been fasting for 24–36 hours a few times a week since then. I have lost another 4 pounds in a few short weeks. My A1C has come down from 5.7 to 5.2 and my fasting blood sugar from 97 to 75 on average. YAY!!! Thank you, thank you, thank you, Jimmy and Dr Fung!!!
>
> **—Robin G.,
> Freeland, MD**

The major problem, as you can see, is not that there aren't enough calories available. There are 350,000 calories stored away in the fat freezer. The problem is that these calories are not available for the body to use. The main issue is how to get access to the energy locked away in the fat. Insulin is the crucial factor to consider here, not the number of calories you eat.

This explains why the *Biggest Loser* contestants, just like all dieters using the "eat less, move more" approach, gained their weight back: their metabolism slowed down in response to caloric reduction. The heavy exercise schedule demanded by the show is also not sustainable for long. Between the slowed metabolism and the reduction in exercise, we see the very familiar weight plateau. Once calorie expenditure drops below intake, we see the even more familiar weight regain. Bam! Goodbye reunion show.

Imagine how this would feel. Reducing your caloric intake by 800 calories per day, as the contestants did, means that you feel cold, lethargic, and tired as your body starts to slow down to conserve energy. After a while, you can't take it anymore. As you increase your calories slightly, you are still eating less than you used to, but because of the slowed metabolism, now you are gaining weight. You return to your original weight as your friends and family silently accuse you of cheating on your diet.

All of this is completely predictable. Since the caloric-reduction strategy has a known 99 percent failure rate, it's no surprise that the *Biggest Loser* strategy has a similarly dismal outlook.

The Solution: Fasting

When we eat, insulin rises and blocks fat-burning, and the body instead burns glucose, which is now freely available from the ingested food. But of the three macronutrients—carbohydrates, fat, and protein—carbohydrates stimulate the production of insulin the most. Refined carbs and sugar in particular have the greatest effect on insulin, so a diet low in these is most certainly a great start for breaking the insulin resistance cycle and losing weight. Yet for some people, this is not enough. Since *all* foods raise insulin levels, the best answer is to completely abstain from food. The answer we are looking for is, in a word, fasting.

Fasting Versus Low-Carb Diets

Both low-carb diets and fasting are able to reduce insulin. So why can't a successful weight-loss strategy be simply eliminating all carbohydrates instead of fasting? It's simply a question of power. Reducing refined carbohydrates reduces insulin. However, protein, especially from animal sources, also raises insulin. Fasting, by restricting everything, keeps insulin lower. Fasting is simply more powerful.

Very low carbohydrate diets (in which carbs compose less than 3 percent of total calories) are very effective at reducing blood sugar in those with type 2 diabetes compared to a standard diet (in which carbs compose 55 percent of total calories). This holds true even when the number of calories consumed is identical. In other words, the glucose-lowering benefits of carb restriction are not simply due to calorie restriction. This is useful knowledge, especially considering how many health professionals insist, "It's all about the calories."

The very low carb diet does remarkably well, providing you 71 percent of the benefits of fasting, without actual fasting. But sometimes low-carb just isn't enough. I've had many patients who limited their carbohydrates but still had elevated blood sugars. How do you get more power? Fasting.

Insulin is the main driver of obesity and diabetes. A very low carb diet can reduce insulin by more than 50 percent, but you can go another 50 percent by fasting. That's power.

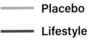

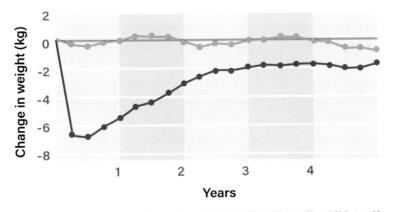

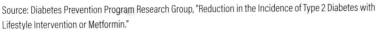

Source: Diabetes Prevention Program Research Group, "Reduction in the Incidence of Type 2 Diabetes with Lifestyle Intervention or Metformin."

Figure 5.10. Weight change over time in the Diabetes Prevention Program, which experimented with preventing diabetes through diet and exercise or medication. Lifestyle changes result in weight loss at first, but eventually the weight returns.

Fasting is simply the most efficient and effective way to lower insulin levels. Notice, however, I did *not* say it was the easiest. But do you want a method that is easy, or a method that works?

Fasting Stops Insulin Resistance When Caloric Reduction Doesn't

There are those who argue that fasting is beneficial only to the extent that it reduces calories. But if that's the case, why is there such a striking difference between caloric reduction and fasting? Caloric-reduction strategies like "eat less, move more" fail virtually every single time, yet fasting is often effective when simple caloric reduction is not. Why?

The short answer is that when you're eating regularly, even if you're eating fewer calories, you're not getting the beneficial hormonal changes of fasting. During fasting, unlike during caloric reduction, metabolism stabilizes or even goes up to maintain normal energy levels. Adrenaline and growth hormone increase to maintain energy and muscle mass. Blood sugar and insulin levels go down as the body changes from burning sugar to burning fat. All this begins to address the long-term problem of insulin resistance.

A recent randomized trial illustrated the difference between the two strategies very well. The study compared the effectiveness of daily caloric reduction and intermittent fasting among 107 women. One group reduced their daily caloric intake from 2,000 calories to 1,500 calories. The other group was allowed normal caloric intake (2,000 calories) five days a week but only 25 percent of that (500 calories) on the remaining two days—this is referred to as a 5:2 fast. This means that over the course of a week, average caloric intake for the two groups was very similar: 10,500 calories per week for the reduced-calorie group and 11,000 calories per week for the fasting group. Both groups consumed similar Mediterranean-style diets with 30 percent fat.

After six months, both groups had similar levels of weight loss and fat loss. But the 5:2 fasting group showed a clear, substantial improvement in insulin levels and insulin resistance, whereas the caloric-reduction group did not.

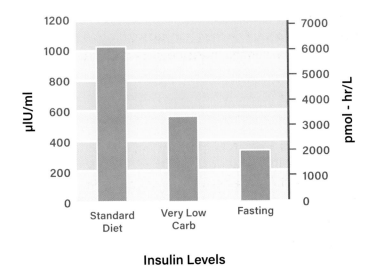

Figure 5.11. A study of type 2 diabetics showed that a very low carb diet does reduce insulin compared to a standard diet, but fasting reduces it even more.

Source: Data from Nuttall et al., "Comparison of a Carbohydrate-Free Diet Vs. Fasting on Plasma Glucose, Insulin and Glucagon in Type 2 Diabetes."

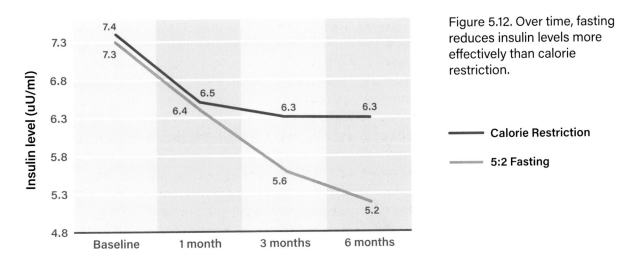

Figure 5.12. Over time, fasting reduces insulin levels more effectively than calorie restriction.

Source: Harvie et al., "The Effects of Intermittent or Continuous Energy Restriction on Weight Loss and Metabolic Disease Risk Markers: A Randomized Trial in Young Overweight Women."

In the long term, this is a crucial problem with caloric reduction. Higher insulin resistance eventually leads to higher insulin levels, which in turn contribute to higher insulin resistance in a vicious cycle. These higher insulin levels inexorably lead to obesity.

The inability of most diets to reduce insulin resistance is exactly why they eventually result in weight regain. Fasting, on the other hand, introduces prolonged periods of low insulin levels, which breaks the cycle of high insulin and insulin resistance.

Another way to look at this is that most diets ignore the biological principle of homeostasis. The body adapts to changing environments. For example, if you are in a dark room and suddenly go into the bright sunlight, you will momentarily be blinded, but within moments your eyes will adapt. The same applies to weight loss. If you maintain a constant reduced-calorie diet, the body will quickly adapt to it. Energy expenditure (metabolism) declines to match the reduced intake. Weight plateaus, then is regained. This is not because you have stopped your diet but because your body has now adapted to it.

To prevent the body from adapting to the new weight-loss strategy and maintain weight loss requires an *intermittent* strategy, not a constant one. This is a crucial distinction. Restricting *some* foods *all* the time differs from restricting *all* foods *some* of the time. This is the difference between failure and success.

ABEL JAMES ◾FASTING ALL-STARS

As a celebrity coach on ABC's *My Diet Is Better Than Yours,* I worked with contestant Kurt Morgan, who began the competition at 352 pounds and 52% body fat. After just 14 weeks following the Wild Diet with intermittent fasting, Kurt lost an astounding 87 pounds. More importantly, Kurt dropped from 52% body fat to less than 30% body fat—nearly doubling the fat loss results of competing dietary approaches. In my experience, combining a high-fat, low-carb nutrition plan with intermittent fasting and strategic strength training can result in rapid and dramatic fat loss.

Bariatric Surgery:
An Argument for Fasting

One intensive weight-loss strategy has proved far more successful than "eat less, move more": bariatric surgery, commonly called "stomach stapling." A study directly comparing *Biggest Loser* contestants—who, you'll recall, used the "eat less, move more" strategy but ultimately regained the weight they lost—to bariatric patients with similar weight loss found that while the contestants experienced metabolic slowdown, the bariatric surgery group did not.

Bariatric surgery is also spectacularly successful for the reversal of type 2 diabetes. In one study, a stunning 95 percent of adolescent patients with type 2 diabetes who underwent bariatric surgery saw their disease reversed. In the same study, after three years, 74 percent saw their high blood pressure resolved and 66 percent saw their abnormal lipids resolved.

Why does bariatric surgery work so well when other diets fail? There have been many theories. The first hypothesis proposed that the removal of most of the healthy stomach produced these benefits. The normal stomach secretes a number of hormones, so the theory went, removing the stomach must reduce some mystery hormone, resulting in the benefits.

This is pretty far-fetched. Newer types of weight loss surgeries, such as gastric banding, involve putting a band around the stomach rather than removing part of the stomach. This kind of surgery is just as successful at reversing type 2 diabetes and reducing insulin resistance. So the benefit cannot be due to the reduction of some mystery hormone secreted by the stomach.

Another thought was that loss of fat cells explained the benefits. Fat cells (adipocytes) actively secrete many different types of hormones, such as leptin, a regulator of body weight. If the fat cells themselves play a role in sustaining obesity, then removal of fat cells would be beneficial. However, liposuction, the mechanical removal of subcutaneous fat, has no metabolic benefit. In one study, the removal of 10 kg (22 pounds) of subcutaneous fat did not significantly improve blood sugars. There was no metabolic improvement, only cosmetic ones.

WHAT HAPPENS WHEN WE BURN FAT: KETONES AND KETOACIDOSIS

You may have heard of a ketogenic diet—it's been quickly growing in popularity in the last several years and is known to be helpful for a wide range of health problems, including obesity. As it happens, a ketogenic diet and fasting have several features in common.

A ketogenic diet gets its name from ketone bodies. These are substances the body produces during fat-burning; they're what fuels the brain when glucose is scarce. A ketogenic diet helps shift the body from burning glucose to burning fat, which results in the creation of ketones. Of course, fasting causes the body to burn fat, too—

and that means it also results in the creation of ketones.

Body fat is composed mostly of triglycerides, which are molecules made of one glycerol backbone to which three fatty acids of varying lengths are attached.

During fat-burning, the triglyceride molecule is broken down into the glycerol backbone and the 3 fatty acids. The fatty acids are used directly by most of the organs of the body, including the liver, kidney, heart, and muscles. However, certain cells are not able to burn fat, including the inner part of the kidney (renal medulla) and red blood cells.

Triglyceride Molecule

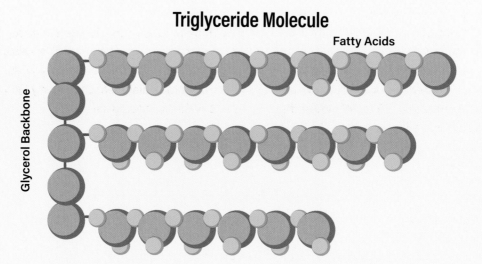

Fatty Acids

Glycerol Backbone

To supply the glucose those cells need, the liver uses the glycerol backbone to manufacture new glucose molecules. More importantly, though, the brain cannot use fatty acids, either. Ketone bodies produced during fat-burning fill that gap, and the brain becomes powered mostly on ketones, which supply up to 75 percent of its energy needs. This dramatically reduces the brain's need for glucose, enabling adequate glucose production from glycerol. In this way, triglycerides provide energy in the form of fatty acids, ketones, and glucose—enough for the entire body. So, yes, the brain still requires glucose to function normally during fasting, but we do not need to *eat* glucose. We can manufacture enough glucose to power the entire body simply from body fat. This is a *normal* situation. This is the way our body is designed to work.

If you have type 1 diabetes, you may have been warned about the dangers of diabetic ketoacidosis. This isn't the same thing as ketosis, which is simply the state of producing ketone bodies. In diabetic ketoacidosis, the body produces ketones even though blood sugar levels are very high.

In this situation, insulin levels *should* be high to handle the blood sugar, but with the insulin-producing pancreatic beta cells destroyed, the body doesn't produce enough insulin. (This is why type 1 diabetics need to take insulin—their bodies simply don't make enough.) Due to the lack of insulin, the body produces lots of ketones. But since there's plenty of glucose in the bloodstream and the brain prefers to use glucose, the ketones are not burned for fuel. Instead they pile up outside cells, like unused logs of firewood. This creates a dangerous, even life-threatening situation.

In the normal, non-diabetic situation, ketones are high but are continuously being burned by the brain for fuel. If you don't have type 1 diabetes, don't worry: you won't develop ketoacidosis!

But there is no real magic or mystery here. Bariatric surgery works because it triggers a sudden and severe caloric reduction. All of the benefits of bariatric surgery are also seen during fasting. Simply put, *bariatric surgery is surgically enforced fasting.*

Bariatric surgery requires patients to dramatically reduce their food intake; eating too much results in nausea and vomiting. This sudden, severe caloric reduction allows the same hormonal adaptations seen during fasting that keep the resting metabolic rate steady, so it doesn't drop as it does when weight is lost due to more gradual, continual caloric reduction. Long-term studies found no decrease in metabolism other than that expected due to the weight loss itself (carrying 300 pounds of weight takes more energy than carrying 200 pounds, so a small slowdown is expected—when we refer to slowing metabolism, we mean the slowdown in excess of that). Adrenaline and growth hormone increase, helping to maintain lean muscle mass and keep metabolism high. Insulin and blood glucose levels fall. The "eat less, move more" strategy for daily caloric reduction doesn't provide these hormonal benefits. However, fasting does.

Head-to-head studies reveal that fasting is actually superior to bariatric surgery in both weight loss and reduction in blood sugars. Both methods are also effective for type 2 diabetes. So here's the crucial question: *If all the benefits of bariatric surgery come from the sudden and severe reduction in calories, why not just fast and skip the surgery entirely?* In essence, fasting is bariatric surgery without the surgery.

There is a price to be paid for any surgery, and with bariatric surgery, complications are common. Within three years of the surgery, 13 percent of adolescent patients had problems severe

MARK SISSON ▮FASTING ALL-STARS▮

Fasting weight loss can often be fleeting because a fair amount of water is lost in the early days (either through a reduction in inflammation from removing offending foods or from the release of glycogen and its stored water). The key to ratcheting down the weight is to not overeat when the fasting period has finished and to maintain a moderate exercise regimen.

enough to require surgery. The most common complication involves scarring that progressively narrows the esophagus, resulting in difficulty eating. To fix this, progressively larger-sized tubes are shoved down the patient's throats to open things up. This procedure is often repeated over and over.

So why not just fast instead? I cannot think of any good reason. The common perception is that if I, as a doctor, recommend cutting out a person's healthy stomach and rewiring their intestines, it's great and I'm serving my patient well, but if I recommend fasting, which accomplishes everything that bariatric surgery does without any complications or costs, then I'm crazy. It's a bizarre conclusion. Fasting is much safer and easier, and its results are just as good, if not better.

Perhaps the most common reason people give for their reluctance to fast is that it is too difficult. Yet, too often, this assessment is made before even *trying* to fast. People say this to me all the time. "I can't fast for twenty-four hours." So I ask them, "How do you know? Have you tried?" To which they answer, "No, I just know that I can't."

In fact, almost everybody *can* fast. There are literally millions of people around the world who regularly fast for religious

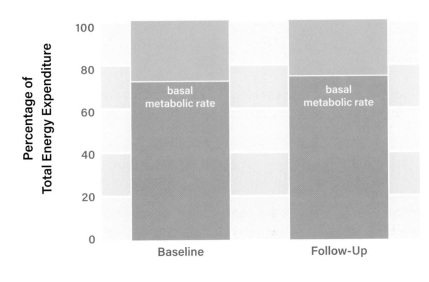

Figure 5.13. Bariatric surgery patients do not show a decrease in their basal metabolic rate, unlike people on simple caloric reduction (see Figure 5.8).

Source: Das et al., "Long-Term Changes in Energy Expenditure and Body Composition After Massive Weight Loss Induced by Gastric Bypass Surgery."

purposes, and before certain blood tests or routine procedures like a colonoscopy, it is standard to fast for up to twenty-four hours. People can fast if they simply try. Like anything else, fasting becomes easier the more often you do it. It doesn't take particular skill—it's not something to do, it's something to *not* do. You simply don't eat. It is subtraction, not addition. This makes it almost the exact opposite of every piece of advice on health ever given (take vitamins, take drugs, have surgery). That's probably why fasting is so successful. To paraphrase *Seinfeld*, everybody wants a show about *something*. This is a show about nothing.

Bariatric surgery certainly has many proven short-term benefits, although long-term benefits are more questionable. *But it's not necessary.* Imagine bariatric surgery without the postoperative complications. Without the cost. Without the need for expensive hospitals or surgical equipment. Without the need for specially trained surgeons. All this is possible with what we might call "medical bariatrics"—fasting.

FASTING AND CORTISOL

Cortisol is a hormone that's released during times of stress, whether physical or psychological. This activates the fight-or-flight response—it's a survival adaptation.

However, cortisol is also one of the major drivers of obesity. In fact, synthetic cortisol, a medication called prednisone, consistently causes weight gain, particularly in the trunk. And because fasting may be considered a potential stressor, some are concerned that it may raise cortisol levels.

But studies of intermittent fasting show that cortisol levels are generally unaffected.

Two weeks of intermittent fasting caused no increase in cortisol levels, and even a seventy-two-hour fast failed to raise cortisol levels significantly. While levels may vary among individuals, on the whole, elevated cortisol levels are not a major concern during fasting. In my experience, the vast majority of people who fast do not have any problem with elevated cortisol levels. However, this does not mean that nobody will ever encounter this problem. On occasion, I have treated patients who felt that fasting negatively affected their cortisol levels. In these cases, it was necessary to change their dietary strategy.

What to Expect When Fasting for Weight Loss

The amount of weight lost on a fasting regimen varies tremendously from person to person. The longer that you have struggled with obesity, the more difficult you'll find it to lose weight. Certain medications, such as insulin, may make it hard to lose weight. You must simply persist and be patient.

You'll probably eventually experience a weight-loss plateau as the weight lost during fasting begins to match the amount regained during eating. (The only way not to plateau at all is to continually fast for weeks or months at a time; otherwise, reaching an equilibrium is inevitable.) Changing either your fasting regimen or diet, or both, may help. Some patients increase fasting from twenty-four-hour periods to thirty-six-hour periods, or try a forty-eight-hour fast. Some try eating only once a day, every day. Others try a continuous fast for an entire week. Any of these can be effective; the key is simply to change the fasting protocol.

Fasting has also been noted to trigger an early period of rapid weight loss, often averaging one to two pounds per day for the first few days. This isn't, unfortunately, due to loss of body fat. Fat loss during fasting averages approximately ½ pound per day. If you are losing 1 pound or more a day, the excess above ½ pound is water weight and will rapidly be regained upon eating. This is not abnormal or unusual. Don't be disappointed when the water weight returns or decide that fasting doesn't work.

References

Albert Stunkard and Mavis McLaren-Hume, "The Results of Treatment for Obesity: A Review of the Literature and Report of a Series," *AMA Archive of Internal Medicine* 103, no. 1 (1959): 79–85.

Alison Fildes, Judith Charlton, Caroline Rudisill, Peter Littlejohns, A. Toby Prevost, and Martin C. Gulliford, "Probability of an Obese Person Attaining Normal Body Weight: Cohort Study Using Electronic Health Records, " *American Journal of Public Health* 105, no. 9 (2015): e54–9. doi:10.2105/AJPH.2015.302773.

Barbara V. Howard, JoAnn E. Manson, Marcia L. Stefanick, Shirley A. Beresford, Gail Frank, Bobette Jones, Rebecca J. Rodabough, et al., "Low-Fat Dietary Pattern and Weight Change over 7 Years: The Women's Health Initiative Dietary Modification Trial," *JAMA* 295, no. 1 (2006): 39–49.

"Best Weight-Loss Diets," *US News & World Report*, n.d., http://health.usnews.com/best-diet/biggest-loser-diet.

Centers for Disease Control, Obesity Prevalence Maps, September 11, 2015, http://www.cdc.gov/obesity/data/prevalence-maps.html.

Christian Zauner, Bruno Schneeweiss, Alexander Kranz, Christian Madl, Klaus Ratheiser, Ludwig Kramer, Erich Roth, Barbara Schneider, and Kurt Lenz, "Resting Energy Expenditure in Short-Term Starvation Is Increased as a Result of an Increase in Serum Norepinephrine," *American Journal of Clinical Nutrition* 71, no. 6 (2000): 1511–5.

Darcy L. Johannsen, Nicolas D. Knuth, Robert Huizenga, Jennifer C. Rood, Eric Ravussin, and Kevin D. Hall, "Metabolic Slowing with Massive Weight Loss Despite Preservation of Fat-Free Mass," *Journal of Clinical Endocrinology and Metabolism* 97, no. 7 (2012): 2489–96.

Diabetes Prevention Program Research Group, "Reduction in the Incidence of Type 2 Diabetes with Lifestyle Intervention or Metformin," *New England Journal of Medicine* 346 (2002): 393–403.

Erin Fothergill, Juen Guo, Lilian Howard, Jennifer C. Kerns, Nicolas D. Knuth, Robert Brychta, Kong Y. Chen, et al., "Persistent Metabolic Adaptation 6 Years After 'The Biggest Loser' Competition," *Obesity* (2016), online May 2, doi: 10.1002/oby.21538.

Frank Q. Nuttall, Rami A. Almokayyad, and Mary C. Gannon, "Comparison of a Carbohydrate-Free Diet Vs. Fasting on Plasma Glucose, Insulin and Glucagon in Type 2 Diabetes," *Metabolism: Clinical and Experimental* 64, vol. 2 (2015): 253–62.

Gina Kolata, "After 'The Biggest Loser,' Their Bodies Fought to Regain Weight," *New York Times*, May 2, 2016, http://www.nytimes.com/2016/05/02/health/biggest-loser-weight-loss.html.

Hodan Farah Wells and Jean C. Buzby, *Dietary Assessment of Major Trends in U.S. Food Consumption, 1970–2005*, US Department of Agriculture: Economic Research Service, Economic Information Bulletin, Number 33, March 2008. http://www.ers.usda.gov/media/210681/eib33_1_.pdf.

Ildiko Lingvay, Eve Guth, Arsalla Islam, and Edward Livingstone, "Rapid Improvement in Diabetes After Gastric Bypass Surgery: Is It the Diet or Surgery?" *Diabetes Care* 36, no. 9 (2013): 2741–7.

J. Gjedsted, L. Gormsen, M. Buhl, H. Nørrelund H, O. Schmitz, S. Keiding, E. Tønnesen, et al., "Forearm and Leg Amino Acids Metabolism in the Basal State and During Combined Insulin and Amino Acid Stimulation After a 3-Day Fast," *Acta Physiologica* 197, no. 3 (2009): 197–205.

John B. Dixon, Paul E. O'Brien, Julie Playfair, Leon Chapman, Linda M. Schachter, Stewart Skinner, Joseph Proietto, et al., "Adjustable Gastric Banding and Conventional Therapy for Type 2 Diabetes," *JAMA* 299, no. 3 (2008): 316–23.

Maarten R. Soeters, Nicolette M. Lammers, Peter F. Dubbelhuis, Mariëtte Ackermans, Cora F. Jonkers-Schuitema, Eric Fliers, Hans P. Sauerwein, et al., "Intermittent Fasting Does Not Affect Whole-Body Glucose, Lipid, or Protein Metabolism," *American Journal of Clinical Nutrition* 90, no. 5 (2009): 1244–51.

Maureen Callahan, "'We're All Fat Again': More 'Biggest Loser' Contestants Reveal Secrets," *New York Post*, January 25, 2015, http://nypost.com/2015/01/25/were-all-fat-again-more-biggest-loser-contestants-reveal-secrets/.

M. N. Harvie, M. Pegington, M. P. Mattson, J. Frystyk, B. Dillon, G. Evans, J. Cuzick, et al., "The Effects of Intermittent or Continuous Energy Restriction on Weight Loss and Metabolic Disease Risk Markers: A Randomized Trial in Young Overweight Women," *International Journal of Obesity* 35, no. 5 (2011): 714–22.

Nicolas D. Knuth, Darcy L. Johannsen, Robyn A. Tamboli, Pamela A. Marks-Shulman, Robert Huizenga, Kong Y. Chen, Naji N. Abumrad, et al., "Metabolic Adaptation Following Massive Weight Loss Is Related to the Degree of Energy Imbalance and Changes in Circulating Leptin," *Obesity* 22, no. 12 (2014): 2563–9.

Roberto A. Ferdman, "One of America's Healthiest Trends Has Had a Pretty Unexpected Side Effect," *Washington Post*, May 24, 2016, https://www.washingtonpost.com/news/wonk/wp/2016/05/24/one-of-americas-healthiest-trends-has-had-a-pretty-unexpected-side-effect/.

Sai Krupa Das, Susan B. Roberts, Megan A. McCrory, L. K. George Hsu, Scott A. Shikora, Joseph J. Kehayias, Gerard E. Dallal, et al., "Long-Term Changes in Energy Expenditure and Body Composition After Massive Weight Loss Induced by Gastric Bypass Surgery," *American Journal of Clinical Nutrition* 78, no. 1 (2003): 22–30.

Samuel Klein, Luigi Fontana, V. Leroy Young, Andrew R. Coggan, Charles Kilo, Bruce W. Patterson, et al., "Absence of an Effect of Liposuction on Insulin Action and Risk Factors for Coronary Heart Disease," *New England Journal of Medicine* 350, no. 25 (2004): 2549–57. doi: 10.1056/NEJMoa033179.

Thomas E. Inge, Anita P. Courcoulas, Todd M. Jenkins, Marc P. Michalsky, Michael A. Helmrath, Mary L. Brandt, Carroll M. Harmon, et al., "Weight Loss and Health Status 3 Years After Bariatric Surgery in Adolescents," *New England Journal of Medicine* 374, no. 2 (2016): 113–23. doi: 10.1056/NEJMoa1506699.

W. J. Pories, K. G. MacDonald Jr., E. J. Morgan, M. K. Sinha, G. L. Dohm, M. S. Swanson, H. A. Barakat, et al., "Surgical Treatment of Obesity and Its Effect on Diabetes: 10-Y Follow-Up," *American Journal of Clinical Nutrition* 55, no. 2 (1992): 582S–585S.

Chapter 6
FASTING FOR TYPE 2 DIABETES

The World Health Organization released its first global report on diabetes in 2016. It's clear from the report that diabetes is an unrelenting disaster. Since 1980, the number of people afflicted with diabetes has quadrupled. How did this ancient disease become the twenty-first century plague?

Diabetes mellitus has been recognized for thousands of years. The ancient Egyptian medical text Ebers Papyrus, written around 1550 B.C., was the first to describe this condition of "passing too much urine." Around the same time, ancient Hindu writings discuss the disease of *madhumeha*, loosely translated as "honey urine." Patients were mysteriously wasting away and no attempt to feed them was successful. Curiously, ants were attracted to their urine, which was inexplicably sweet. By 250 B.C. Greek physician Apollonius of Memphis had termed the condition *diabetes*, which by itself connotes excessive urination. How is it possible that this disease of antiquity could dominate our current health-care system despite all the advances in medicine, technology, and nutrition of the past few thousand years?

There are two main types of diabetes, type 1 and type 2. In many ways these two are opposites of one another. Type 1 diabetes is an autoimmune disease. For unknown reasons, the body's own immune system attacks and destroys the insulin-producing cells in the pancreas, leading to a severe insulin deficiency.

Type 2 diabetes, on the other hand, is a dietary and lifestyle disease. In response to frequent high blood sugar, the body produces excessive insulin, which leads to insulin resistance—just as we stop being able to smell a particular odor in a room after a while, the body stops being able to respond to insulin's signals after prolonged exposure to excess insulin. There is a clear association between type 2 diabetes and obesity, and weight loss often reverses this type of diabetes.

Because type 1 diabetics lack insulin, for them, insulin injections are a life-saving treatment. However, in the case of type 2 diabetes, giving insulin to patients is not particularly successful—after all, their bodies are already making plenty of insulin (too much, in fact). For them, dietary therapies hold the most promise of success. The history of dietary therapies for type 2 diabetes goes back several centuries, but unfortunately, the lessons of the past have largely been forgotten.

Early Treatments for Diabetes

Up until the mid-nineteenth century, no specific treatments were available for either type of diabetes. Type 1 diabetes was uniformly fatal until the discovery of insulin in 1921. Type 2 diabetes was quite uncommon until the twentieth century, for two reasons: first, it is typically diagnosed after age fifty (in fact, it used to be called adult-onset diabetes) and average life expectancy was lower than it is today, and second, food was not nearly as available and plentiful. The combination of relative food scarcity and low average life expectancy meant that type 2 diabetes was rare, and little effort was expended to search for effective treatments. It was generally accepted that diabetes was a uniformly fatal disease without any specific or effective treatment.

This changed when Apollinaire Bouchardat (1806–1886), sometimes called the founder of modern diabetology, established a therapeutic diet for diabetes based upon his observation that during the Franco-Prussian War, periodic starvation resulted in less urinary glucose excretion. His book *De la Glycosurie ou Diabète Sucré* (*Glycosuria or Diabetes Mellitus*) lays out his comprehensive dietary strategy, which forbade foods such as sugars and starches. This is eerily similar to the low-carbohydrate diets that have recently been recognized, once again, to be effective in the treatment of type 2 diabetes.

LCHF got me halfway, fasting got me the rest of the way! I've fixed the insulin resistance that I've had for 20 years, and I'm now down 30 pounds. I'm a US size 4 at 40 years old. Amazing!

—Claire,
Adelaide, Australia

At the turn of the twentieth century, prominent American physicians Frederick Madison Allen (1879–1964) and Elliott Joslin (1869–1962) became the leading proponents of intensive dietary therapy for diabetes. Allen envisioned diabetes as a disease where the "overstrained" pancreas could no longer keep up with the demands of an excessive diet. This idea does not stray far from our current understanding of the "burned-out" pancreas in type 2 diabetes. Allen's hypothesis was that a severely reduced diet would reduce the workload for the dysfunctional pancreas enough that it could cope. Patients could thus survive until the pancreas completely failed.

Allen's "starvation treatment" was widely considered the best therapy (dietary or otherwise) until the discovery of insulin in 1921. This diet was very low in calories (800 per day) and very restricted in carbohydrates (less than 10 grams per day). Patients were admitted to hospital and treated with whiskey and black coffee every two hours from 7 a.m. to 7 p.m.; they abstained from all other foods. (It's unclear why Dr. Allen thought whiskey was necessary.) This continued until sugar disappeared from the urine. After this induction phase, low-carbohydrate foods were gradually reintroduced into the diet, along with protein, as long as the glucose in the urine remained low. This draconian restriction on foods resulted in many reports of adults weighing only 65 pounds. Nevertheless, the response of some diabetics was stunning, unlike anything seen previously. The symptoms of excessive urination and thirst, caused by the glucose in the urine, often improved significantly.

Allen published his first case series of forty-four patients in 1915 in the *American Journal of the Medical Sciences*. Between 1914 and 1917, he treated a further ninety-six patients with an average admission of sixty-nine days, the longest being 304 days. There was no shortage of physicians ready to refer their "hopeless" diabetics to Allen. However, it is unclear whether patients continued to follow such a Spartan dietary regimen once discharged from the hospital. Allen published detailed clinical results of seventy-six patients in his 1919 book *Total Dietary Regulation in the Treatment of Diabetes*.

It is highly likely that the patients who responded so well to Allen's treatment were, in fact, suffering from type 2 diabetes or incomplete type 1 diabetes. However, the usefulness of Allen's treatment was severely hampered by the lack of understanding of the differences between type 1 and type 2 diabetes. Type 1 diabetic patients were often severely underweight children while type 2 diabetic patients were mostly overweight adults, and the ultra-low-calorie diet could be deadly for the severely malnourished type 1 diabetics. In fact, many children starved to death on this diet, which Allen and Joslin euphemistically called *inanition*, a term that technically refers to exhaustion due to starvation. It was a tragic outcome, but keep in mind that since type 1 diabetes was almost uniformly fatal, Allen and Joslin were trying a last-ditch strategy to save their lives. It was widely understood, even by Allen, that his treatment was only a desperate trade-off between death from diabetes and death from starvation and malnutrition. Nevertheless, it represented the first viable treatment for diabetes and, as such, was a major advance. The Allen diet became standard treatment in many academic medical centers and is widely acknowledged to have saved the lives of hundreds or thousands of patients by allowing them to live long enough to herald the development of insulin injections.

Joslin, the first American doctor to specialize in diabetes and likely the most famous diabetologist in history, founded the world-famous Joslin Diabetes Center in Boston and wrote the authoritative textbook *The Treatment of Diabetes Mellitus*, which is still in publication today. He found that Allen's treatments brought significant, almost miraculous improvements in some of his patients and wrote in 1916, "That temporary periods of under-nutrition are helpful in the treatment of diabetes will probably be acknowledged by all after these two years of experience with fasting."

In 1921, Frederick Banting and John Macleod discovered insulin at the University of Toronto. There was widespread euphoria in the belief that diabetes had finally been cured, and all interest in dietary treatments was effectively terminated. But unfortunately, the story of diabetes does not end there. It was only a false spring.

While insulin rescued type 1 diabetics from the brink of death, it did little to improve the overall condition of type 2 diabetics. Luckily, in the early twentieth century, type 2 diabetes was still a rare disease, as was obesity. However, by the late 1970s, the rate of obesity had started its relentless march upwards. Ten years later, type 2 diabetes started its own inexorable increase.

Over the past thirty years, the rate of type 2 diabetes has increased significantly in both sexes, in every age group, in every racial and ethnic group, and at all education levels. It is attacking younger and younger patients: pediatric diabetes clinics, once the sole domain of type 1 diabetes, are now overrun with an epidemic of type 2 diabetes, often in obese adolescents.

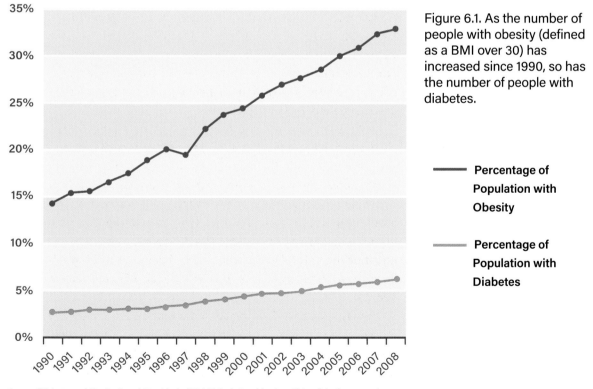

Figure 6.1. As the number of people with obesity (defined as a BMI over 30) has increased since 1990, so has the number of people with diabetes.

—— Percentage of Population with Obesity

—— Percentage of Population with Diabetes

Source: "Diabetes and Obesity Growth Trend in the U.S.," *Diabetic Care*, blog, http://blog.diabeticcare.com/diabetes-obesity-growth-trend-u-s/. Data from cdc.gov.

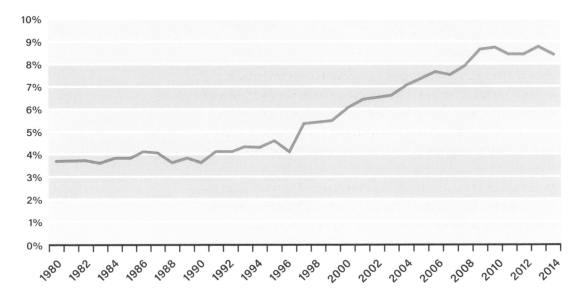

Figure 6.2. The percentage of Americans with diabetes has grown steadily since 1980, and the rate of the increase rose sharply in the late 1990s.

Source: Data from cdc.gov.

Despite the explosion of medical advances and knowledge since the 1800s, ironically, diabetes is an even bigger problem today than it was then. In the nineteenth century and before, diabetes was a rare, though frequently fatal, disease. Fast-forward to 2016, and there are more Americans with prediabetes and diabetes than without: in 2012, 14.3 percent of American adults had diabetes and 38 percent had prediabetes, for a total of 52.3 percent. Diabetes is increasing in every corner of the world. Almost all these patients are overweight and will suffer complications related to their diabetes. It's one of the world's oldest diseases, but where the incidence of most other diseases has improved over time with advancing medical knowledge, diabetes is getting worse, to the point that we now have a worldwide epidemic.

But *why*? Why are we powerless to stop the spread of type 2 diabetes?

Forgotten Wisdom: The Relationship Between Type 2 Diabetes and Diet

Today, diabetes specialists consider type 2 diabetes to be a chronic and progressive disease. However, bariatric surgery, which reduces stomach size to severely restrict food intake, proves that this is not true. Type 2 diabetes very often improves within a few weeks of this surgery, even before massive amounts of weight are lost.

As we discussed in Chapter 5, both fasting and bariatric surgery result in a sudden, severe restriction of foods, so it's not surprising that fasting has a similar effect. In fact, it's been known to cure type 2 diabetes for over a hundred years. Joslin thought the truth of it was so obvious that studies were not even needed. Interestingly, visceral fat, fat that's stored in and around the organs, likely plays a large role in type 2 diabetes. It's more harmful to health and, unfortunately, more common than subcutaneous fat. Fasting and bariatric surgery both preferentially reduce visceral fat.

Consider, for example, the effect of wartime starvation on type 2 diabetes. During both World War I and World War II, the mortality rate from type 2 diabetes dropped precipitously. This was due to wartime food rationing, which resulted in a sustained, severe reduction of calories. Figure 6.3 shows the co-occurrence of wartime sugar rationing and a drop in deaths from diabetes, but

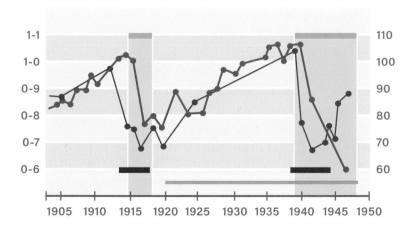

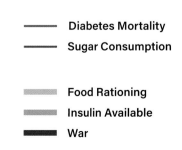

Figure 6.3. Diabetes mortality improved during wartime rationing.

— Diabetes Mortality
— Sugar Consumption

▨ Food Rationing
▨ Insulin Available
▬ War

Source: Cleave, *The Saccharine Disease.*

keep in mind that it wasn't just sugar that was rationed—almost all foods were restricted, resulting in a sustained, severe calorie reduction similar in magnitude to Fredrick Allen's infamous starvation diet.

Consider these weekly rations for an adult in the United Kingdom during World War II:

Bacon	4 oz
Sugar	8 oz
Tea	2 oz
Cheese	2 oz
Butter	2 oz

I think my thirteen-year-old son would eat through these weekly rations in a single meal and still ask for dessert!

Interestingly, diabetics were forced to surrender their sugar rations completely and given butter instead. In the interwar period, as people went back to their accustomed eating habits, the mortality rate went back up, even though insulin injections were introduced as a treatment for diabetes in the early 1920s.

US ration books from World War II.

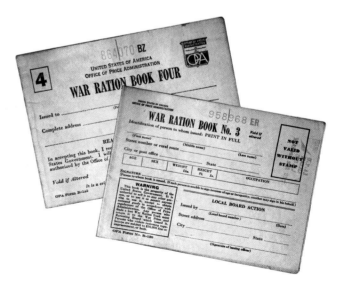

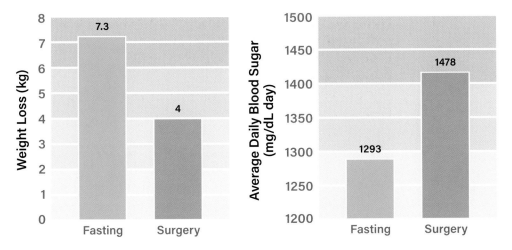

Source: Lingvay, "Rapid Improvement in Diabetes After Gastric Bypass Surgery: Is It the Diet or Surgery?"

Figure 6.4. Fasting results in better weight loss and blood sugar levels than bariatric surgery.

A study comparing fasting and bariatric surgery revealed that fasting is perhaps even more beneficial in the treatment of type 2 diabetes. In a head-to-head comparison, fasting lowered both body weight and blood sugar better than bariatric surgery.

These results show that, rather than the chronic and progressive disease it's often seen as, type 2 diabetes is a treatable and reversible condition. This changes everything.

Why Fasting Works for Type 2 Diabetes

It is well known and well accepted that type 2 diabetes is a disease of insulin resistance. One of insulin's main jobs is to move glucose from the blood into the tissues, which use it as energy. When insulin resistance develops, the normal level of insulin is not able to move glucose into tissue cells. Why?

Let's consider an analogy. Imagine the cell to be a subway train. Glucose molecules are the passengers waiting to get inside the train. Insulin gives the signal to open the train doors, and the passengers—the glucose molecules—march in a nice orderly manner into the empty subway train. Normally, it doesn't really require much of a push to get this glucose into the cell.

Figure 6.5. A model of insulin resistance: when a cell is overfilled with glucose, it appears resistant to insulin's signals to allow more glucose to enter.

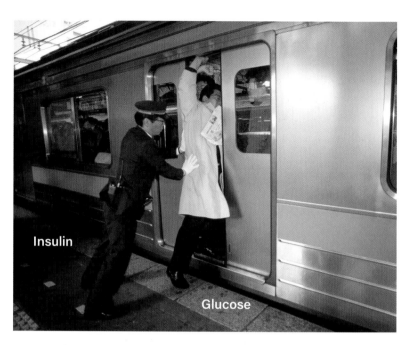

Insulin

Glucose

By utilizing Dr. Fung's advice on fasting, I was able to come off insulin and just take metformin. I find now that if I fast for 20 to 23 hours per day—basically only eat dinner—I can get by without taking my metformin. I find I feel better if I maintain this schedule of fasting.

—Laura K., Nashville, TN

But what happens if the train is not empty? What if it's already jam-packed full of passengers? Insulin gives the signal to open the door, but the passengers waiting on the platform cannot enter. From the outside, it appears that this train (cell) is now resistant to insulin's signals.

So, what can you do to pack more people into the train? One solution is to hire subway pushers to shove people into the trains. This was implemented in New York City in the 1920s, and while the practice has since died out in North America, subway pushers still exist in Japan, where they are euphemistically called "passenger arrangement staff."

Insulin is the body's subway pusher, shoving glucose into the cell no matter the consequences. If the normal amount of insulin can't get the glucose in, then the body calls for reinforcements: even more insulin. But the main cause of the insulin resistance is that the cell was already overflowing with glucose.

Because the cell is overfilled with glucose, glucose spills out of the cell, leading to increased blood glucose levels. This leads to the diagnosis of type 2 diabetes. If you now give more insulin, or drugs that stimulate the production of insulin, then yes, temporarily, more glucose can be shoved into the cell. However, there is a natural limit. At that point, even extra insulin will not be able to move more glucose into the cell.

This is exactly what happens in the typical time course of type 2 diabetes. At first, the disease can be treated with a small dose of a single medication that stimulates the production of insulin. After a few years, this is no longer enough, so the dose is increased. After a few more years, a second, then a third medication is added, all aimed at increasing the production of insulin. Finally, insulin itself is prescribed in higher and higher doses. The progression of treatments is clearly not helping the underlying problem: the type 2 diabetes is just getting worse. The medications only help control blood sugar; they don't address what's causing type 2 diabetes.

If the core issue is that glucose is overfilling the cells, then the solution seems rather obvious: get all that glucose out of the cells! Pushing more in, as with insulin treatments, will only make things worse. So how do you get rid of excess glucose in the body? (Remember, it's the glucose in the tissue cells that's the underlying problem—without that, the glucose in the bloodstream is no longer a problem.)

There are really only two methods of getting the toxic glucose overload out of the body. First, you need to stop putting glucose into the body. You can achieve this with very low carbohydrate diets or ketogenic diets. Indeed, many people have reversed their diabetes by following such diets. Fasting also eliminates carbohydrates—and all other foods, for that matter.

Second, your body needs to burn off the excess glucose. Fasting is again an obvious solution. Your body requires energy just to keep all the vital organs, such as the heart, lungs, liver, and kidneys, working. Your brain in particular requires substantial energy to function properly, even during sleep. During fasting, no new glucose is coming in, so your body has no choice but to use up the stored glucose.

At its core, type 2 diabetes is a disease of excessive glucose, in our blood but also in our bodies. If you don't eat, your blood sugar level will come down. Once your blood sugars are consistently in the normal range, you will no longer be considered diabetic. Presto! Diabetes reversed. Mischief managed.

Extended fasting has lowered my morning (upon awakening) blood sugar to an all-time low of 4.7. Never in my 15 years as a diabetic have I ever experienced this exceptional number.

—Liliana D.,
Toronto, ON

Careful Monitoring Is Essential

If you are on medications for type 2 diabetes or any other conditions, then it is imperative that you speak with your physician before embarking on the fasting journey. Most diabetic medications work to lower blood sugar based on your current diet. If you change your diet without adjusting your medications, then there is a real risk of having low blood sugar, which is extremely dangerous. You may feel shaky, sweaty, or nauseated. In more severe cases, it may cause loss of consciousness and even death. Therefore, it is essential that you discuss any planned dietary changes with your physician so he or she can monitor you and adjust your medications as necessary.

Most medications unrelated to blood sugar can be taken during fasting, though you should still discuss them with your physician first. If you are not taking any blood sugar medications, then there is no particular reason to monitor your blood sugar during fasting: your blood sugar may drop slightly but will remain in the normal range.

However, if you are taking medication for diabetes—and again, be sure you talk to your physician before fasting!—then it's essential to frequently monitor your blood sugar. You should check your blood sugar at least twice a day and ideally up to four times a day on both fasting and nonfasting days. Certain medications are more prone to causing hypoglycemia (low blood sugar) than others, and your physician will be able to guide you.

I often advise patients to reduce or avoid their blood sugar medications during fasting days and to only take them when blood sugar goes too high. If they are a little high, it is not often a

AMY BERGER FASTING ALL-STARS

One of the benefits of fasting is that it helps very strongly insulin-resistant/hyperinsulinemic people finally tap into their stored body fat for energy—plus there are the myriad other benefits that come from reducing insulin levels. After decades of metabolic dysregulation, some people really have to pull out all the stops to get their insulin levels back into a healthy range, and fasting helps many accomplish this.

problem, since you are not eating and can expect it to come down a little without intervention. However, if they become too high, taking a dose of medication will bring it back down. I consider the optimal blood sugar range while fasting to be 8.0 to 10.0 mmol/L, if you are taking medication. This range is higher than the nonfasting norm, but the mildly elevated levels are not harmful in the short term while we are attempting to improve the diabetes, and the primary goal while you're fasting and still on blood sugar medication is to avoid dangerous hypoglycemia events. The long-term goal is to successfully wean yourself off medications and maintain sugars in the normal range.

It is generally better to use less medication during fasting. If your blood sugar goes higher than you wish, you can always take more medication to compensate. However, if your blood sugar goes too low, you must eat some sugar. That will break the fast and is counterproductive to reversing the diabetes. Again, consult with your doctor before you try fasting for your type 2 diabetes.

References

Allan Mazur, "Why Were 'Starvation Diets' Promoted for Diabetes in the Pre-Insulin Period?" *Nutrition Journal* 10, no. 23 (2011), doi: 10.1186/1475-2891-10-23.

Andy Menke, Sarah Casagrande, Linda Geiss, and Catherine C. Cowie, "Prevalence of and Trends in Diabetes Among Adults in the United States, 1988-2012," *JAMA* 314, no. 10 (2015): 1021–9, doi:10.1001/jama.2015.10029.

Elliot P. Joslin, *The Treatment of Diabetes Mellitus* (Philadelphia: Lea & Febiger, 1916).

Elliot P. Joslin, "The Treatment of Diabetes Mellitus," *Canadian Medical Association Journal* 6, no. 8 (1916): 673–84.

Frederick Allen, "Prolonged Fasting in Diabetes," *American Journal of Medical Sciences* 150 (1915): 480–5.

Frederick M. Allen, Edgar Stillman, and Reginald Fitz, *Total Dietary Regulation in the Treatment of Diabetes* (New York: Rockefeller Institute for Medical Research, 1917).

"Frederick Allen," *Diapedia: The Textbook of Diabetes* (website), August 13, 2014, http://dx.doi.org/10.14496/dia.1104519416.6.

Ildiko Lingvay, Eve Guth, Arsalla Islam, and Edward Livingstone, "Rapid Improvement in Diabetes After Gastric Bypass Surgery: Is It the Diet or Surgery?" *Diabetes Care* 36, no. 9 (2013): 2741–7.

T. L. Cleave, *The Saccharine Disease* (Bristol, UK: John Wright & Sons Limited, 1974).

MEGAN

FASTING SUCCESS STORY

My name is Megan, and I am the director of Dr. Fung's Intensive Dietary Management Program in Toronto. Actually, I'm not only the IDM Program director; I'm also a patient! In fact, I was the program's very first patient.

Like most of our patients, I have struggled with my weight and health over the years. When I was younger I could eat my weight in Chicken McNuggets every day without gaining a pound. At twenty-three, I only weighed ninety-seven pounds and ate more than a frat boy. I didn't have problems maintaining my weight or staying healthy, but my mother always warned me things would go downhill at thirty-five. As it turned out, it happened even sooner.

Just after my twenty-sixth birthday, I suddenly gained fifty-three pounds over a period of four months. That year was the worst year of my life. I was drowning in personal turmoil and felt like I was sinking in quicksand. During this time period I sought comfort in food, particularly McNuggets—and it showed. As the year progressed, I became less depressed about my personal life and more depressed about my physical appearance.

I had no energy to do anything and experienced constant brain fog. I stopped caring about almost everyone and everything. I couldn't get up for work in the morning. I showed up places looking like I was homeless.

Knowing that things needed to change, I adopted a strict low-fat, calorie-restricted diet, limiting myself to 800 calories and less than 15 grams of fat per day. I ate five or six times throughout the day and worked out for an hour five times a week. In the first two weeks, I lost twelve pounds. But over the following four weeks, I only lost a pound per week. After that, the weight loss stopped altogether, despite my best efforts. In fact, I started to gain back some of the weight I had lost.

I could not figure out why I wasn't losing weight. I might not have been eating the healthiest of foods, but I wasn't eating very much, either. Carefully tracking my caloric intake revealed that I was only consuming 1461 calories and 41 grams of fat each day. How was I gaining weight? I was stumped.

I went to see a very prominent and expensive dietitian in Toronto. After reviewing my food list, she said I had been making excellent choices. Her best advice? I should exercise more. Five hours of exercise a week was not enough? I went to the gym every morning and evening for the next two weeks, but my weight did not budge. The next time I went back to see the dietitian, she rolled her eyes at me. I knew she thought I was lying. Her advice? Try harder. That was the last time I saw her.

I was beyond frustrated. I felt defeated. Eating six small meals daily, I never felt full. I was constantly obsessing over food. Not long after, I was diagnosed with a heart condition and an early stage of a rare cancer believed to be related to my aspartame addiction. Bloodwork also revealed that my HbA1c—a marker of blood glucose—had climbed up to 6.2 percent. I was now prediabetic.

Having worked as a medical researcher since I was eighteen years old, I was well aware of the damage that type 2 diabetes can do. I literally watched diabetes destroy people's health every day. Kidney failure, nerve damage, blindness, heart attacks, strokes—I had seen it all. I was petrified.

Just at this time, my colleague Dr. Fung was developing the Intensive Dietary Management Program to help people reverse their diabetes and obesity, based upon a deeper understanding of the core problem.

The truth about obesity, insulin, and diabetes was almost the total opposite of everything I had learned in university about nutrition. But it made total sense. At last, I understood why I could not lose weight and had developed prediabetes. Better, I knew exactly what I needed to do about it.

Fasting

I won't lie to you—I was scared to try fasting. The first fasting day was very difficult, and I struggled for the first two weeks. On my first attempt to do a twenty-four-hour fast, I only lasted for twenty-two hours. But I told myself that twenty-two hours was still a great success. After all, that was twenty-two hours longer than I had ever fasted before. I wasn't even hungry by the end of the twenty-two hours. I didn't need to eat—I just wanted to. That was when I truly knew that fasting is mind over matter.

I reached the twenty-four-hour mark successfully on my second fasting day. Staying busy was the key. I went to the gym that evening thinking I was going to fall off of the spin bike. But hey, I figured there were enough people there to save me if that happened. Incredibly, exercise was actually a lot easier while fasting!

Each fasting day got easier. At first I did experience headaches, but a few cups of good homemade bone broth with sea salt did the trick. After a month, the headaches were a thing of the past. My energy levels started to increase. After two months of fasting, I was able to increase the duration of my fast to thirty-six hours without difficulty. Nowadays, I will occasionally add a seven-day fast as well, and my longest fast was fourteen days. There are days I actually feel better fasting.

I also struggled with the idea of a high-fat diet. Growing up, I was told bacon was reserved for patients in palliative care. We never ate whole eggs, just egg whites. Avocados were banned, and I don't ever remember seeing butter in the house, only margarine. It took a while for me to adjust to the idea of eating more natural fats, but the more I ate, the better the results.

Reducing carbs was not easy, either. I experienced headaches, nausea, and tremors despite normal blood sugar and pressure readings. I would sit in my car during lunch breaks because I felt like I was withdrawing from heroin and the walls were closing in. I was scared to go into a shopping mall and be surrounded by fast food. I felt like the McDonald's drive-thru was trying to pull my car in. I would avoid certain routes on my daily commute. Was I going insane? I found that eating more natural fats helped. I started taking tablespoons of coconut oil and eating half of an avocado on my eating days.

Results

Within three months of starting my plan, I'd lost thirty-three pounds and reached my target weight. A few months later, I had lost sixty pounds, and I maintained that weight for over a year and a half without difficulty. In fact, I lost another fifteen pounds of unhealthy fat without trying, and put on ten pounds of lean muscle tissue besides.

My hemoglobin A1c in March 2016 was 4.7 percent, having remained under 5.0 percent since February 2013. I have never felt so good or been in better shape. Previously, I had taken medication for ADHD while attempting certain tasks, but now I don't need anything. I have never been able to focus so well in my life!

I still enjoy holidays and indulge on special occasions, but I have learned how to balance my diet. If I indulge myself on a vacation, I balance this by fasting more when I come home. I went to a San Francisco Giants game on Sunday and had a Ghirardelli sundae. I tell all of my patients to have one if they are ever in San Francisco. My weight was up dramatically on Monday, but I didn't panic—I knew that most of it was water weight. I fasted on Monday, drinking a lot of water and adding some coconut oil into my tea in the morning. I had no headaches. I didn't feel nauseous. My weight was back down to my pre-sundae weight by Tuesday morning. Life is all about finding a balance. Feast and fast. It has been easy for me to maintain my weight loss and health since.

Intensive Dietary Management Program

My experiences have enabled me to help our patients achieve their own health goals. I have done a lot of self-experimentation over the years, and there is not anything I ask of our patients that I have not tried myself. And I'm constantly learning from our patients each and every day.

Every individual has a different experience with fasting. Everyone has different challenges. We work together with the patient to find out what works. Some patients prefer to fast for days at a time rather than on alternate days. Sometimes patients have panic attacks thinking about fasting for more than a day. I help patients find out what works best for their lifestyle. I coach the patients on their fasting and troubleshoot any issues that arise. I help patients work up to achieving longer periods of fasting, just as I had to do. We adjust the duration and frequency of fasts depending on their goals and progress.

Nutrition is an important aspect of the program. Our goal is to try to limit how much insulin the body needs to produce each day. This is easy during fasting days because the body will only produce the amount of insulin required to function normally. However, this presents a bit of a challenge on eating days. I help transition patients to a high-fat, moderate-protein, and low-carbohydrate diet. Most people are just as perplexed as I was about what they can eat once carbohydrates are drastically reduced. Let me reassure you, there are many great foods that you can indulge in that will leave you completely satiated. I've learned to enjoy eggs in a thousand different ways. I eat chicken wings and bacon regularly. You can eat bacon and eggs guilt-free because you know you are doing something really good for your body! It sounds really weird, I know.

Most of our IDM patients have type 2 diabetes or prediabetes. Nonalcoholic fatty liver disease, sleep apnea, and polycystic ovary syndrome are common. We offer two different programs to our patients: our in-office clinic and our long-distance program. I coach patients in both programs on how to fast and what and when to eat. Our in-office program treats patients from across Canada. Sometimes they will do the long-distance program in between office visits. We will see patients weekly, biweekly, or monthly for their duration in our program. Our long-distance program allows me to connect with people all over the world and offer them the same advice and patient education.

The long-distance program has helped further diversify my knowledge about food and nutrition among a variety of different cultures. Just this morning I was able to speak to a woman in Sweden and a man in Singapore. We have patients in France, New Zealand, Australia, South Africa, India, China, the United Kingdom, and throughout various parts of North America.

It has been such an honor to watch the transformations in my patients. For the first time in my career I get to watch people get better. Almost every time a patient comes to see us, they are a little bit better than the time before. It is the most incredible feeling to witness this firsthand. I am so proud and grateful to work with such an amazing group of patients, who work so hard and are so dedicated to achieving a healthier lifestyle.

Chapter 7
FASTING FOR A YOUNGER, SMARTER YOU

The most obvious benefits of fasting are that it helps with weight loss and type 2 diabetes, but there are many other benefits, including autophagy (a cellular cleansing process), lipolysis (fat-burning), anti-aging effects, and neurological benefits. In other words, fasting can benefit your brain and help your body stay younger.

Boosting Brainpower

Mammals generally respond to severe caloric deprivation by reducing organ size, with two prominent exceptions: the brain and, in males, the testicles. Reproductive function is preserved to propagate the species. But cognitive function is just as important and also highly preserved, at the expense of every other organ.

This makes a lot of sense from an evolutionary standpoint. Suppose food is scarce and difficult to find. If cognitive function started to decline, the mental fog would make it that much harder to find food. Our brainpower, one of the main advantages we have in the natural world, would be squandered. So what actually happens during caloric deprivation is that the brain maintains or even boosts its abilities. The best-selling novel *Unbroken*, by Laura Hillenbrand, describes the experiences of American prisoners of war in Japan during World War II. During their extreme starvation, the prisoners experienced some astonishing mental clarity that

Originally, I was interested in the fasting research that demonstrated a reduction in inflammation and increase in growth hormone. However, when I began fasting through the morning, I immediately noticed a significant increase in mental focus, energy, and productivity. As a brain science geek, I'm impressed by the mental benefits of fat-adaptation and intermittent fasting.

they themselves understood was due to the effect of starvation. One man was able to learn Norwegian in just under a week. Another described "reading" entire books from memory.

Humans, like all mammals, have an increase in mental activity when hungry and a decrease when satiated. We have all experienced a "food coma"— think about how you feel after a big Thanksgiving meal, complete with turkey and pumpkin pie. Are you mentally sharp as a tack? Or dull as a concrete block? Despite popular belief, it's not the tryptophan in the turkey causing that postprandial drowsiness—in fact, turkey has about the same amount of tryptophan as other poultry. It's just the sheer amount of food. As the amount of blood going to the digestive system is increased to handle all that turkey and pie, less blood is available to go to the brain. About the only mental challenge we can handle after that enormous meal is sitting on the couch watching football.

How about the opposite? Think about a time that you were really, really hungry. Were you tired and sluggish? I doubt it. You were probably hyperalert, your senses sharp as a needle. Animals that are cognitively sharp and physically agile during times of food scarcity have a clear advantage when it comes to survival. If missing a single meal reduced our energy and mental acuity, we would have even more trouble finding food, making it more likely that we would go hungry again, leading to a vicious cycle ending in death. That's not, of course, what happens. Our ancient ancestors grew more alert and active when hungry so that they could find their next meal—and the same thing still happens to us.

I am a 58-year-old woman. I intermittent fast almost daily for 16–18 hours. I find that I have more energy to get through a workout in a fasted state. I also have better mental clarity.

—Diane Z., Chicago, IL

Even our language reflects the relationship between hunger and mental acuity. When we say we are hungry for something—hungry for power, hungry for attention—does it mean we are slothful and dull? No, it means that we are on our toes, alert and ready for action. Fasting and hunger energize us and activate us to advance towards our goal, despite popular misconceptions to the contrary.

In one study of mental acuity and fasting, none of the factors measured—including sustained attention, attentional focus, simple reaction time, and immediate memory—were found to be impaired. Another study of two days of almost total caloric deprivation found no detrimental effect on cognitive performance, activity, sleep, and mood.

That's what happens to our brains during fasting. But the neurological benefits of fasting aren't limited to the times when we're actually forgoing food. Animal studies show that fasting has remarkable promise as a therapeutic tool. Aging rats started on intermittent fasting regimens markedly improved their motor coordination, cognition, learning, and memory. Interestingly, there was even increased brain connectivity and new neuron growth from stem cells. A protein called brain-derived neurotrophic factor (BDNF), which supports the growth of neurons and is important for long-term memory, is believed to be responsible for some of these benefits. In animals, both fasting and exercise significantly increase the beneficial BDNF effects in several parts of the brain. Compared to normal mice, mice on an intermittent fasting regimen showed less age-related deterioration of neurons and fewer symptoms of Alzheimer's disease, Parkinson's disease, and Huntington's disease.

Human studies on caloric reduction find similar neurologic benefits—and since fasting certainly restricts calories, this is one area where fasting and caloric reduction provide similar benefits. With a 30 percent reduction in calories consumed, memory significantly improved and the synaptic and electrical activity in the brain increased.

In addition, insulin levels have an inverse correlation to memory—that is, the lower the insulin level, the more memory improves. On the flip side, a higher body mass index is linked to

I've spent 6 months doing alternate-day fasting as well as periodic 1–5 day fasts. The first day is the hardest, but I feel so focused on fasting days, it is worth it!

—Scott J., Minneapolis, MN

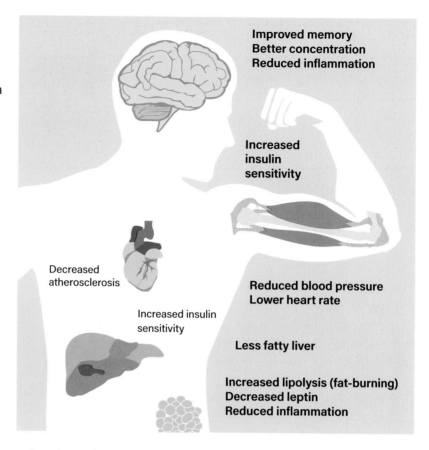

Figure 7.1. The multiple beneficial effects of fasting on various parts of the body.

Improved memory
Better concentration
Reduced inflammation

Increased insulin sensitivity

Decreased atherosclerosis

Reduced blood pressure
Lower heart rate

Increased insulin sensitivity

Less fatty liver

Increased lipolysis (fat-burning)
Decreased leptin
Reduced inflammation

Source: Longo and Mattson, "Fasting: Molecular Mechanisms and Clinical Applications."

decline in mental abilities and decreased blood flow to those areas of the brain involved in attention, focus, reasoning, and more complex, abstract thought. So fasting provides neurological benefits two ways: it decreases insulin and leads to consistent, maintained weight loss.

Slowing Aging

When you buy a new car, everything works great. But after a few years, it starts to get a little beat up and needs more maintenance. You need to replace the brake pads, then the battery, then more and more parts. Eventually, the car is breaking down all the time and costing thousands of dollars to maintain. Does it make sense to keep it around? Likely not. So you get rid of it and buy a snazzy new car.

There appears to be significant research indicating a dramatic drop in inflammation, improvements in insulin signaling, and a near total "reset" of immune function with fasts of 3–5 days. Abnormal and or pre-cancerous cells appear to be pushed towards apoptosis, which essentially selects for healthy cell types. In total this describes a process which should (in theory) reverse many of the signs and symptoms of aging while reducing the processes that appear to be at play in autoimmunity and cancer.

In this sense, the cells of the body are like cars. As they age, subcellular parts need to be removed and replaced, and eventually, a cell gets too old to repair and needs to be destroyed to make way for a healthy new cell.

In a process called apoptosis, also known as programmed cell death, cells that reach a certain age are programmed to commit suicide. While this may sound kind of macabre at first, the process constantly renews cell populations, making it essential for good health. But when just some cellular components need to be replaced, a process called autophagy kicks in.

The word *autophagy*, coined by Nobel Prize–winning scientist Christian de Duve, derives from the Greek *auto* ("self") and *phagein* ("to eat"). So the word literally means "to eat oneself." Autophagy is a form of cellular cleansing: it is a regulated, orderly process of breaking down and recycling cellular components when there's no longer enough energy to sustain them. Once all the diseased or broken-down cellular parts have been cleansed, the body can start the process of renewal. New tissues and cells are built to replace those that were destroyed. In this way, the body renews itself. But it only works if the old parts are discarded first.

Our bodies are in a constant state of renewal. While we often focus on new cell growth, we sometimes forget that the first step in renewal is destroying the old, broken-down cellular machinery. But apoptosis and autophagy are both necessary to keep our bodies running well. When these processes are hijacked, diseases such as cancer occur, and the accumulation of older cellular components may be responsible for many of the effects of aging. These unwanted cellular components build up over time if autophagocytic processes are not routinely activated.

Increased levels of glucose, insulin, and proteins all turn off autophagy. And it doesn't take much. Even as little as 3 grams of the amino acid leucine can stop autophagy. Here's how it works: The mammalian target of rapamycin (mTOR) pathway is an important sensor of nutrient availability. When we eat carbohydrates or protein, insulin is secreted, and the increased insulin levels, or even just the amino acids from the breakdown of ingested protein, activate the mTOR pathway. The body senses that food is available and decides that since there's plenty of energy to go around, there's no need to eliminate the old subcellular machinery. The end result is the suppression of autophagy. In other words, the constant intake of food, such as snacking throughout the day, suppresses autophagy.

Conversely, when mTOR is dormant—when it's not being triggered by increased insulin levels or amino acids from ingested food—autophagy is promoted. As the body senses the temporary absence of nutrients, it must prioritize which cellular parts to keep. The oldest and most worn-out cellular parts get discarded, and amino acids from the broken-down cell parts are delivered to the liver, which uses them to create glucose during gluconeogenesis. They may also be incorporated into new proteins. It's important to note that the dormancy of mTOR is only related to short-term nutrient availability and not the presence of stored energy, such as liver glycogen or body fat. Whether the body has stored energy is irrelevant for mTOR and therefore for autophagy.

AMY BERGER ▮ FASTING ALL-STARS

For people with chronic inflammatory and/or neurological conditions, fasting can help accelerate autophagy and the body's clearing-out of old, damaged tissue. The body engages in "housecleaning" all the time, but when it gets a break from the constant digestion of large amounts of food, it may be able to focus more energy on repair and restoration.

This is why the strongest stimulus to autophagy currently known is fasting, and why fasting alone, unique among diets, stimulates autophagy—simple caloric restriction or dieting isn't enough. By eating constantly, from the time we wake up to the time we sleep, we prevent the activation of autophagy's cleansing pathways. Simply put, fasting cleanses the body of unhealthy or unnecessary cellular debris. This is the reason longer fasts were often called cleanses or detoxifications.

At the same time, fasting also stimulates growth hormone, which signals the production of some new snazzy cell parts, giving our bodies a complete renovation. Since it triggers both the breakdown of old cellular parts and the creation of new ones, fasting may be considered one of the most potent anti-aging methods in existence.

Autophagy also plays an important role in the prevention of Alzheimer's disease. Alzheimer's is characterized by the abnormal accumulation of amyloid beta (Aß) proteins in the brain, and it's believed that these accumulations eventually destroy the synaptic connections in the memory and cognition areas. Normally, clumps of Aß protein are removed by autophagy: the brain cell activates the autophagosome, the cell's internal garbage truck, which engulfs the Aß protein targeted for removal and excretes it, so it can be removed by the blood and recycled into other protein or turned into glucose, depending upon the body's needs. But in Alzheimer's disease, autophagy is impaired and the Aß protein remains inside the brain cell, where eventual buildup will result in the clinical syndromes of Alzheimer's disease.

Cancer is yet another disease that may be a result of disordered autophagy. We're learning that mTOR plays a role in cancer

FASTING ALL-STARS — DR. THOMAS SEYFRIED

Fasting can limit growth of glucose-dependent tumors. Fasting can also target inflammation that contributes to the initiation and progression of tumors. We showed that fasting or calorie restriction could significantly reduce distal tumor invasion in our preclinical models of brain cancer.

biology, and mTOR inhibitors have been approved by the Food and Drug Administration for the treatment of various cancers. Fasting's role in inhibiting mTOR, thereby stimulating autophagy, provides an interesting opportunity to prevent cancer's development. Indeed, some leading scientists, such as Dr. Thomas Seyfried, a professor of biology at Boston College, have proposed a yearly seven-day water-only fast for this very reason.

References

Anne M. Cataldo, Corrinne M. Peterhoff, Juan C. Troncoso, Teresa Gomez-Isla, Bradley T. Hyman, and Ralph A. Nixon, "Endocytic Pathway Abnormalities Precede Amyloid β Deposition in Sporadic Alzheimer's Disease and Down Syndrome," *American Journal of Pathology* 157, no. 1 (2000): 277–86.

Anne M. Cataldo, Deborah J. Hamilton, Jody L. Barnett, Peter A. Paskevich, and Ralph A. Nixon, "Properties of the Endosomal-Lysosomal System in the Human Central Nervous System: Disturbances Mark Most Neurons in Populations at Risk to Degenerate in Alzheimer's Disease," *Journal of Neuroscience* 16, no. 1 (1996): 186–99.

A. V. Witte, M. Fobker, R. Gellner, S. Knecht, and A. Flöel, "Caloric Restriction Improves Memory in Elderly Humans," *Proceedings of the National Academy of Sciences of the United States of America* 106, no. 4 (2009): 1255–60.

Danielle Glick, Sandra Barth, and Kay F. Macleod, "Autophagy: Cellular and Molecular Mechanisms," *Journal of Pathology* 221, no. 1 (2010): 3–12.

Erin L. Glynn, Christopher S. Fry, Micah J. Drummond, Kyle L. Timmerman, Shaheen Dhanani, Elena Volpi, and Blake B. Rasmussen, "Excess Leucine Intake Enhances Muscle Anabolic Signaling But Not Net Protein Anabolism in Young Men and Women," *Journal of Nutrition* 140, no. 11 (2010): 1970–6.

Harris R. Lieberman, Christina M. Caruso, Philip J. Niro, Gina E. Adam, Mark D. Kellogg, Bradley C. Nindl, and F. Matthew Kramer, "A Double-Blind, Placebo-Controlled Test of 2 D of Calorie Deprivation: Effects on Cognition, Activity, Sleep, and Interstitial Glucose Concentrations," *American Journal of Clinical Nutrition* 88, no. 3 (2008): 667–76.

Helena Pópulo, Jose Manuel Lopes, and Paula Soares, "The mTOR Signalling Pathway in Human Cancer," *International Journal of Molecular Sciences* 13, no. 2 (2012): 1886–1918.

Kristen C. Willeumier, Derek V. Taylor, and Daniel G. Amen, "Elevated BMI Is Associated with Decreased Blood Flow in the Prefrontal Cortex Using SPECT Imaging in Healthy Adults," *Obesity* 19, no. 5 (2011): 1095–7.

Mark P. Mattson, "Energy Intake and Exercise as Determinants of Brain Health and Vulnerability to Injury and Disease," *Cell Metabolism* 16, no. 6 (2012): 706–22.

Melanie M. Hippert, Patrick S. O'Toole, and Andrew Thorburn, "Autophagy in Cancer: Good, Bad, or Both?" *Cancer Research* 66, no. 19 (2006): 9349–51.

Michael W. Green, Nicola A. Elliman, Peter J. Rogers, "Lack of Effect of Short-Term Fasting on Cognitive Function," *Journal of Psychiatric Research* 29, no.3 (1995): 245–53.

Noboru Mizushima, "Autophagy: Process and Function," *Genes & Development* 21, no. 22 (2007): 2861–73.

Per Nilsson, Krishnapriya Loganathan, Misaki Sekiguchi, Yukio Matsuba, Kelvin Hui, Satoshi Tsubuki, Motomasa Tanaka, Nobuhisa Iwata, Takashi Saito, and Takaomi C. Saido, "Aβ Secretion and Plaque Formation Depend on Autophagy," *Cell Reports* 5, no. 1 (2013): 619–69.

Valter D. Longo and Mark P. Mattson, "Fasting: Molecular Mechanisms and Clinical Applications," *Cell Metabolism* 19, no. 2 (2014): 181–92.

Zhineng J. Yang, Cheng E. Chee, Shengbing Huang, and Frank A. Sinicrope, "The Role of Autophagy in Cancer: Therapeutic Implications," *Molecular Cancer Therapeutics* 10, no. 9 (2011): 1533–41.

Chapter 8
FASTING FOR HEART HEALTH

A little starvation can really do more for the average sick man than can the best medicines and the best doctors.

—Mark Twain

High blood cholesterol is classically considered a treatable risk factor for cardiovascular disease, including heart attacks and strokes. That's led to a popular conception of cholesterol as some kind of poison, but this is far from the truth. Cholesterol is used to repair cell walls and also to make certain hormones. It is so vital for human health that virtually every cell in the body has the ability to manufacture cholesterol if needed.

Traditionally, blood tests measure low-density lipoprotein (LDL), or "bad," cholesterol, and high-density lipoprotein (HDL), or "good," cholesterol. Cholesterol travels in the bloodstream bundled together with proteins, which are then called lipoproteins. Which lipoproteins are associated with the cholesterol molecule determines whether the bundle is LDL or HDL—the cholesterol molecule itself is the same.

What we call "high cholesterol" refers to LDL cholesterol, and large epidemiological studies have associated increased levels of LDL with increased risk of cardiovascular disease. Certain drugs, particularly statins, can significantly reduce the levels of LDL. But what caused it to go up in the first place? This question still has no satisfactory answer. However, the initial hypothesis was that it must be a dietary problem. Turns out, as we'll explore in a moment, that's not the case.

Another risk factor for heart disease is a type of fat called triglycerides. When glycogen stores in the liver are full, the liver starts converting excess carbohydrates into triglycerides instead. These triglycerides are then exported out of the liver as very low density lipoprotein (VLDL). VLDL is used to form LDL.

High levels of triglycerides in the blood are strongly associated with cardiovascular disease. It is almost as powerful a risk factor as high LDL cholesterol, which is what doctors and patients tend to be more concerned about. Higher blood triglyceride levels, independent of LDL, increase the risk of heart disease by as much as 61 percent. This is concerning because the average triglyceride level has been rising inexorably in the United States since 1976, along with type 2 diabetes, obesity, and insulin resistance. An estimated 31 percent of adult Americans are currently estimated to have elevated triglyceride levels, paralleling the rise in consumption of carbohydrates.

Fortunately, high triglycerides can be treated with a low-carbohydrate diet, which lowers the rate at which the liver creates triglycerides. But while triglyceride levels respond to diet, the same cannot be said for cholesterol.

High Cholesterol Isn't a Dietary Problem

If eating too much dietary cholesterol caused blood cholesterol levels to go up, then it would be reasonable to assume that eating less cholesterol would lower blood cholesterol levels. And over the last three decades, health-care professionals have exhorted people to reduce their dietary cholesterol intake by eating fewer high-cholesterol foods, such as egg yolks and red meat. The USDA's *Dietary Guidelines for Americans*, from its very inception, stated quite clearly that we should "avoid too much fat, saturated fat, and cholesterol."

Unfortunately, this idea is entirely wrong. The scientific community has long known that eating less cholesterol does not lower blood cholesterol. Our liver generates 80 percent of the cholesterol found in the blood, so eating less cholesterol makes little or no difference. By the same token, eating more cholesterol does not raise blood cholesterol significantly. If we eat less dietary cholesterol, our liver simply compensates by creating more, so

> I do IF every other day, about 20 hours. I have absolutely no problems finishing my workouts or other activities. I have found the biggest thing it has helped with is my digestion. I am way more regular now, and I also can also go longer between meals. In one year I also improved my triglycerides from 135 to 100 and raised my HDL a couple points to 60.
>
> —Brian W., Dayton, OH

the net effect is negligible. Furthermore, it's not the cholesterol particle itself that's cause for concern—remember, that's identical in both LDL and HDL. It's instead the lipoproteins carried along with the cholesterol particle that determine whether it's good or bad. Reducing the cholesterol in our foods makes little or no physiological difference, a fact that was proven long ago.

Our irrational fear of dietary cholesterol began in 1913. Atherosclerotic plaques, the blockages in the arteries that cause heart attacks and strokes, are predominantly composed of cholesterol, and it was hypothesized that these plaques were caused by too much dietary cholesterol. This makes as much sense as supposing that eating beef heart will make your own heart stronger, but then, this was 1913. That year, Russian scientist Nikolai Anichkov discovered that feeding cholesterol to rabbits caused atherosclerosis. Rabbits, however, are herbivores and aren't meant to eat foods that contain cholesterol. Feeding a lion hay would also cause health problems. Unfortunately, this fundamental fact was not appreciated in the rush to find a culprit for the plaques.

Ancel Keys confirmed that dietary cholesterol was not a problem as early as the 1950s. One of the preeminent nutritional researchers of his era, he fed human subjects increasing amounts of cholesterol to see if there was any resulting increase in blood cholesterol levels. There was not. His Seven Countries Study, one of the largest epidemiological studies of diet and nutrition ever done, also established that eating cholesterol does not raise blood cholesterol.

As dietary cholesterol was acquitted, dietary fat became the prime suspect—perhaps, the thinking went, high dietary intake of fat somehow leads to increased cholesterol levels. This, too, has long been disproven, primarily by the Framingham studies. In 1948, the residents of Framingham, Massachusetts, were enrolled in a long-term study that followed all aspects of their lifestyles, including diet, to establish what factors are important in the development of heart disease. It is still running strong, now with its third generation of participants. Thousands of medical papers have been written about the Framingham Heart Study, but history has virtually forgotten the Framingham Diet Study.

The original Framingham study.

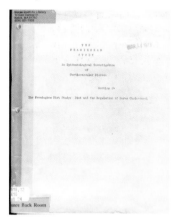

This ambitious study, which ran from 1957 to 1960 and involved over one thousand participants, attempted to find a connection between dietary fat and blood cholesterol—which researchers already believed existed. After millions of dollars and years of painstaking observation, exasperated researchers failed to discover any discernable correlation between dietary fat and blood cholesterol levels. Whether people ate a lot of fat or very little fat made no difference to cholesterol.

These findings clashed vigorously with the prevailing conventional wisdom, and researchers were presented with a choice. They could accept these results and search for a nutritional theory closer to the truth, or they could simply ignore them and continue to believe what had just been proven false. Unfortunately, they took the latter choice. The results were tabulated and then quietly suppressed and never published in a peer-reviewed journal. Dissenters to nutritional orthodoxy, no matter how correct, were not to be tolerated.

Decades later, Dr. Michael Eades tracked down a lost copy of this important study. The statistician Tavia Gordon lamented, "Unfortunately, these data were never incorporated into a definitive report by the original investigators and a large amount of very careful and thoughtful work has lain unused in the Framingham files." The study found that "there is a slight negative association between daily intake of total fat (and also of animal fat) with serum cholesterol level." In other words, the more dietary fat eaten, the lower blood cholesterol. And a local newspaper article from the town of Framingham in 1970 plainly stated, "There is no discernable relationship between reported diet intake and serum cholesterol levels in the Framingham Diet Study group."

But the low-fat religion prevailed, and healthy high-fat foods such as nuts, avocados, and olive oil were incriminated for decades. But the truth cannot be suppressed forever, and other studies went on to confirm that dietary fat does not raise cholesterol.

The link between dietary fat and cholesterol was also studied in the community of Tecumseh, Michigan, in 1976. The population was divided into three groups based on blood cholesterol levels—low, medium, and high. The dietary habits of each group were

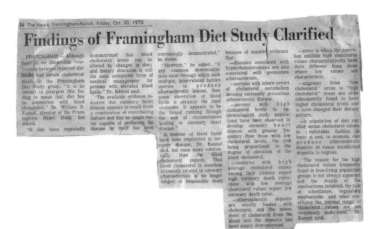

A 1970 article in the Framingham-Natick *News* pointed out that the Framingham Diet Study showed no relationship between diet and blood cholesterol levels.

Source: Dr. Michael Eades.

compared, and to the researchers' surprise, each group ate identical amounts of fat, animal fats, saturated fats, and cholesterol. Once again, it was clear that eating fat did not raise blood cholesterol.

Another study fed one group of volunteers a diet that was 22 percent fat and a second group a diet that was 39 percent fat. Baseline cholesterol for both groups was 173 mg/dl. After fifty days, the cholesterol levels in the low-fat group plummeted to . . . 173 mg/dl. Oh. High-fat diets don't raise cholesterol much, either. After fifty days, cholesterol levels in the high-fat group increased only marginally, to 177 mg/dl.

Even following a very strict low-fat diet has no beneficial effects on blood cholesterol. In one study, LDL did decrease marginally by 5 percent, but HDL also decreased by 6 percent—since both "bad" and "good" cholesterol dropped, the overall risk profile was not improved.

Despite all the evidence to the contrary, national dietary guidelines in the United States and United Kingdom were introduced in 1977 and 1983 recommending adhering to a low-fat diet in order to reduce the risk of heart disease. A careful meta-analysis and systematic review by Zoe Harcombe confirmed that there was no evidence that these recommendations would be effective, either at the time of publication or today.

I've been practicing the 16:8 IF protocol and eating a low-carb, high-fat diet between 10 a.m. and 6 p.m. on most days. About once a month I kick it into high gear with an extended 40-hour "fat fast" consisting of sparkling water, coffee with butter, cream, and MCT oil, and a little bone broth. As a result, I've lost about 40 pounds in 4 months, with dramatically improved lipids and glucose markers.

**—Robert H.,
Walnut Creek, CA**

Millions of people follow a low-fat, low-cholesterol diet because they think that it's good for their heart, without realizing that these measures were long ago proven ineffective. Frank Hu and Walter Willett of the Harvard School of Public Health wrote in 2001, "It is now increasingly recognized that the low-fat campaign has been based on little scientific evidence and may have caused unintended health consequences." So, does this mean that the only reliable way to lower blood cholesterol is to take drugs? Hardly. There is one simple, natural measure that lowers cholesterol: fasting.

Why Fasting Lowers Cholesterol

The liver produces the vast majority of cholesterol found in the blood. Eating less cholesterol has almost no effect on the liver's production. In fact, it may be counterproductive. As the liver senses less incoming cholesterol, it may simply increase its own production.

So why does fasting affect the liver's production of cholesterol? As dietary carbohydrates decline, the liver decreases its synthesis of triglycerides—since excess carbohydrates are converted

Figure 8.1. Alternate-day fasting reduces LDL cholesterol.

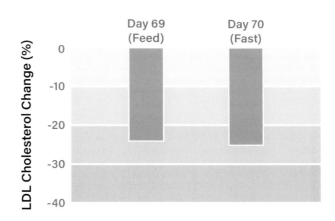

Source: Bhutani et al., "Improvements in Coronary Heart Disease Risk Indicators by Alternate-Day Fasting Involve Adipose Tissue Modulations."

to triglycerides, the absence of carbohydrates means fewer triglycerides. Remember that triglycerides are released from the liver as VLDL, which is the precursor of LDL. Therefore, reduced VLDL eventually results in lowered LDL.

The only reliable way to reduce LDL levels is to reduce the liver's production of it. In fact, studies prove that seventy days of alternate-day fasting could reduce LDL by 25 percent. This is far in excess of what can be achieved with almost any other diet and about half of the effect achieved with a statin medication, one of the most powerful cholesterol-reducing medications available. Triglyceride levels drop by 30 percent, similar to what can be achieved with a very low carbohydrate diet or medication. Not bad for an all-natural, cost-free dietary intervention.

Plus, whereas statins carry the risk of diabetes and Alzheimer's disease, fasting reduces body weight, preserves fat-free mass, and decreases waist circumference. In addition, fasting preserves HDL, unlike low-fat diets, which tend to decrease both LDL and HDL. Overall, fasting produces significant improvements in multiple cardiac risk factors. For people worried about heart attacks and strokes, the question is not "Why are you fasting?" but "Why are you *not* fasting?"

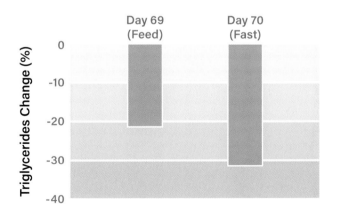

Figure 8.2. Alternate-day fasting reduces triglyceride levels.

Source: Bhutani et al., "Improvements in Coronary Heart Disease Risk Indicators by Alternate-Day Fasting Involve Adipose Tissue Modulations."

References

A. B. Nichols, C. Ravenscroft, D. E. Lamphiear, and L. D. Ostrander Jr., "Daily Nutritional Intake and Serum Lipid Levels. The Tecumseh Study," *American Journal of Clinical Nutrition* 29, no. 12 (1976): 1384–92.

Ancel Keys, "Atherosclerosis: A Problem in Newer Public Health," *Journal of Mount Sinai Hospital New York* 20, no. 2 (1953): 118–39.

F. Hu, J. Manson, and W. Willet, "Type of Dietary Fat and Risk of Coronary Heart Disease: A Critical Review," *Journal of the American College of Nutrition* 20, no. 1 (2001): 5–19.

Gary J. Nelson, Perla C. Schmidt, and Darshan S. Kelley, "Low-Fat Diets Do Not Lower Plasma Cholesterol Levels in Healthy Men Compared to High-Fat Diets with Similar Fatty Acid Composition at Constant Caloric Intake," *Lipids* 30, no. 11 (1995): 969–76.

Gregory G. Schwartz, Markus Abt, Weihang Bao, David DeMicco, David Kallend, Michael Miller, Hardi Mundi, and Anders G. Olsson, "Fasting Triglycerides Predict Recurrent Ischemic Events in Patients with Acute Coronary Syndrome Treated with Statins," *Journal of the American College of Cardiology* 65, no. 21 (2015): 2267–75.

Igor E. Konstantinov, Nicolai Mejevoi, and Nikolai M. Anichkov, "Nikolai N. Anichkov and His Theory of Atherosclerosis," *Texas Heart Institute Journal* 33, no. 4 (2006): 417–23.

Michael Eades, "Framingham Follies," *The Blog of Dr. Michael R. Eades, M.D.*, September 26, 2006, https://proteinpower.com/drmike/2006/09/26/framingham-follies/.

Michael Miller, Neil J. Stone, Christie Ballantyne, Vera Bittner, Michael H. Criqui, Henry N. Ginsberg, Anne Carol Goldberg, et al., "Triglycerides and Cardiovascular Disease: A Scientific Statement from the American Heart Association," *Circulation* 123, no. 20 (2011): 2292–333.

R. L. Rosenthal, "Effectiveness of Altering Serum Cholesterol Levels Without Drugs," *Proceedings* (Baylor University Medical Center) 13, no. 4 (2000): 351–5.

Surabhi Bhutani, Monica C. Klempel, Reed A. Berger, and Krista A. Varady, "Improvements in Coronary Heart Disease Risk Indicators by Alternate-Day Fasting Involve Adipose Tissue Modulations," *Obesity* 18, no. 11 (2010): 2152–9.

Zoë Harcombe, Julien S. Baker, Stephen Mark Cooper, Bruce Davies, Nicholas Sculthorpe, James J. DiNicolantonio, and Fergal Grace, "Evidence from Randomised Controlled Trials Did Not Support the Introduction of Dietary Fat Guidelines in 1977 and 1983: A Systematic Review and Meta-analysis," *Open Heart* 2, no. 1 (2015): e00196, doi: 10.1136/openhrt-2014-000196.

Chapter 9
WHAT YOU NEED TO KNOW ABOUT HUNGER

I have discussed the therapeutic use of fasting for obesity and type 2 diabetes with hundreds of patients over the years. Most, if not all, people understand fundamentally why this treatment is undeniably effective: If you don't eat, you will lose weight. If you don't eat, your blood sugar will decrease. Yet, almost universally, there is still an initial, severe resistance to the idea of even attempting to incorporate fasting into their lives. Why? One fear stands like a colossus above all others: hunger.

Without a doubt, uncontrollable hunger is the most common worry about fasting. Even some "experts" proclaim (incorrectly!) that this will leave you prone to severe overeating once the fast is over. They say, "Don't miss a single meal, otherwise you will be so hungry that you will be forced to stuff your face full of Krispy Kreme donuts." And most people worry that they will simply be unable to continue fasting because they will be overwhelmed with hunger.

Somewhat surprisingly, practical experience with hundreds of patients shows that while they're on an intermittent fasting regimen, they most often see their hunger *diminish*, not increase. They often report that despite their own expectations, they are eating less than half their usual amount of food on a daily basis, yet they feel completely full. For most people, this is the most pleasant surprise of fasting.

> The first three days, I was clamoring for something to chew and was consuming many cups of bone broth to make the feeling go away. On the fourth day, it did—all was well. I have used fasting to lose the last 10 pounds that was too stubborn to leave me, and now I do a monthly fast for weight maintenance and insulin control.
>
> **—Gloria M., Washington, DC**

We start to feel hunger pangs approximately four hours after our last meal. So we imagine that fasting for a full twenty-four hours creates hunger sensations six times stronger—and that would be intolerable. But this does *not* happen. Overcoming hunger often seems a daunting task, but that stems from a fundamental misunderstanding about the nature of hunger.

Hunger Starts in the Mind

We often believe that hunger is simply a natural physiological reaction to not eating, as inevitable as a rainstorm. We have a mental image that as our stomach fills up with food, it signals our brain that we are full. We imagine that as our stomach empties and drops below a critical threshold, our brain signals us to eat. That is not the entire truth. Consider how hungry you feel first thing in the morning. Studies of circadian rhythm confirm that for most people, hunger is very low first thing in the morning, even though it has been twelve to fourteen hours since the last meal. Conversely, hunger at dinnertime is often very high, even though we have often eaten lunch just a mere six hours ago.

Hunger, obviously, is not simply a reflection of the amount of food filling our stomach. Instead, hunger is partly a learned phenomenon. Even when we don't think we're hungry, smelling a steak and hearing it sizzle may make us quite ravenous. These kinds of food-related stimuli do not need to be learned; they're innate in almost everyone. But we can also learn to become hungry during conditions that are intrinsically unrelated with food. For example, the sound of a dinner bell can create hunger where it had not previously existed. The power of these stimuli was demonstrated by the classic experiments of Pavlov's dogs.

In the 1890s, the Russian scientist Ivan Pavlov was studying salivation in dogs. Dogs salivate when they see food and expect to eat. This reaction occurs naturally and without training. In his experiments, lab assistants fed the dogs, and the dogs soon began to associate lab coats with eating. There is nothing intrinsically appetizing about a man in a lab coat, but because the dogs consistently were fed by a lab-coat-wearing man, the lab coat and food became paired in the dogs' minds.

Soon the dogs began to salivate at the sight of the lab coats alone, even if food was not present. Ivan Pavlov, genius that he was, noticed this association, and before you know it, he was packing his bags to Stockholm to receive his Nobel Prize.

The applicability of this Psychology 101 lesson to hunger is obvious. We can become hungry for many reasons. Some stimuli naturally make us hungry, such as the smell and sizzle of steak. Other stimuli need to be consistently associated with food in order to provoke hunger on their own.

These conditioned responses can be very powerful. In fact, there are measurable physical reactions to the mere suggestion of food. Salivation, pancreatic fluid secretion, and insulin production increase immediately upon the *expectation*, not the actual delivery, of food. This helps synchronize the gut response and the incoming food, and is known as the cephalic phase response.

The reason great restaurants spend so much time and energy on plating food is because they understand that our enjoyment does not begin with the first bite—it begins when we see the food. An attractively plated meal makes us hungrier than the same food slopped haphazardly into a dog dish. Hunger, in this case, starts with the eyes. But there are infinite other possible associations with foods that make us hungry.

If we consistently eat every morning at 7:00 a.m., then we develop a conditioned response to that time and become hungry at 7:00 a.m., even if we ate a huge meal at dinner the night before. The same applies to lunch and dinnertime. We become hungry merely because of the time, not any true intrinsic hunger. This is learned only through decades of association. Children, on the other hand, often refuse food early in the morning because they are simply not hungry.

Similarly, by consistently pairing movies with delicious popcorn and sugary drinks, the mere thought of a movie may make us hungry. Food companies, of course, spend billions of dollars trying to condition us to make these associations. Food at the ball game! Food at the movies! Food while watching TV! Food in between halves at our kids' soccer games! Food while listening to a lecture! Food at a concert! Conditioned responses, every one. The possibilities are endless.

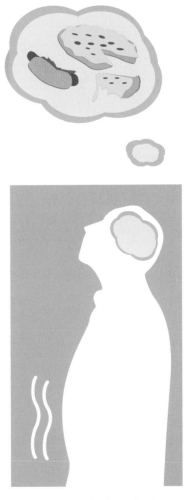

Hunger starts in the mind.

There is a coffee shop or fast food restaurant on every corner. There are vending machines in every nook and cranny of every building in North America. And if we start salivating like Pavlov's dog every four hours simply because the clock says it's time to eat, and we're conditioned to associate the sight of the golden arches with eating, it is little wonder we find it increasingly difficult to resist McDonald's. We are bombarded daily with images of and references to food. The combination of their convenience and our ingrained Pavlovian response is deadly and fattening. How can we fight this?

Defeating Hunger Conditioning

Intermittent fasting offers a unique solution. By randomly skipping meals and varying the intervals at which we eat, we can break our habit of eating three times a day, come hell or high water. We no longer have a conditioned response of hunger every three to five hours. We no longer become hungry simply because it's noon or we're at the movies. That's not to say we don't get hungry at all—we do, but not simply because we have a conditioned response to a certain time or occasion. Instead, we *get hungry because we are hungry*. We allow our body to tell us when it needs nourishment rather than eating by the clock.

Have you ever been so busy at work or school that you simply forgot to eat breakfast and lunch? You were simply too focused on

AMY BERGER ▮FASTING ALL-STARS

For most people, the biggest obstacles to fasting are psychological, rather than physiological. In the modern industrialized world, we are accustomed to eating 'round the clock. We eat when we're happy, sad, bored, excited, stressed out, lonely, watching television, celebrating, and just about anything and everything else. In order to fast successfully, try to divorce yourself from the notion that you are "supposed to" eat several times a day. It is okay—beneficial, in fact—to become reacquainted with feelings of hunger. In fact, it's actually kind of nice to get reacquainted with the signals our bodies send us . . . when we finally allow them to come through. We are wired for feast and famine, not feast, feast, feast.

the task at hand to heed any of the numerous hunger cues. Your body just used some of the plentiful energy stored as body fat as fuel.

Here's the simplest way to break associations between food and anything else: Eat only at the table. No eating at your computer station. No eating in the car. No eating on the couch. No eating in bed. No eating in the lecture hall. No eating at the ball game. Try to avoid mindless eating—every meal should be enjoyed as a meal, not as something eaten while watching a movie. In this way, food becomes associated only with the kitchen and the table. These are not new ideas, of course; it was just common sense in your grandmother's generation.

But in breaking habits, going cold turkey is not often successful. Instead, it is better to replace one habit with another, less harmful habit. This is, of course, the reason that people who are trying to quit smoking often chew gum. If your habit is to eat munchies while watching television, simply stopping will make you feel like something is missing. Instead, replace that snacking habit with a habit of drinking a cup of herbal or green tea. Yes, this may seem weird at first, but you will feel a lot less like something is missing. Ultimately, swapping one habit for another is a far more successful strategy.

It's also helpful to avoid artificial sweeteners. Even though they contain no calories, they may still kick off the cephalic phase response, stimulating hunger as well as insulin production. I don't recommend artificial sweeteners during fasting for this very reason. Recent studies confirm that diet sodas are generally not helpful for weight loss, probably because they trigger hunger but don't satisfy it.

FASTING ALL-STARS ABEL JAMES

Fasting can be a powerful tool to recalibrate your relationship with eating habits and perceived hunger. True hunger is generally experienced in the body and brain, not in the stomach. It may take some practice, but once you reconnect with the feeling of true hunger, you can follow your body's lead and eat whenever the feeling strikes.

Handling Hunger Conditioning During Fasting

Our conditioned response to feel hunger at certain stimuli and the cephalic phase response mean that there are certain things we can do to make fasting easier. Of course, there are many natural stimuli to hunger that cannot entirely be abolished. However, following some simple rules will make hunger much easier to handle.

First, as mentioned above, artificial sweeteners can kick off the cephalic phase response, triggering hunger and insulin production, so I recommend avoiding them during a fast. There are certainly people who feel that adding sweeteners to their coffee helps them lose weight by increasing compliance with their fast, and if it works for you, great. But my best advice is to try to fast without the use of sweeteners. If you cannot do that, then try adding a small amount. However, if it makes fasting harder or prevents you from seeing results, then stop.

Second, try to physically remove yourself from all food stimuli during a fast. Cooking a meal or even just seeing and smelling food while fasting is almost unbearably difficult. This is not simply a matter of weak willpower. Our cephalic phase responses are fully activated, and to feel those responses without actually eating is like trying to stop a piranha feeding frenzy. This, of course, is the same reason you should not shop for food when hungry, or keep snacks in the pantry.

Simply breaking the habit of eating at certain times can be difficult. One thing you can try is to make a habit of drinking a large cup of coffee or tea along with breakfast on nonfasting days. On fasting days, you will still miss the food, but having your daily cup of joe will make it easier to not eat—you won't be avoiding the habit of consuming something in the morning. You can also have a bowl of homemade bone broth at dinnertime on fasting days. It makes fasting easier in the long run.

One of our most important tips for fasting is to *stay busy*. Working through lunch and staying busy means I often don't even remember to be hungry. My cephalic phase response has not been activated. If somebody were to put food in front of me, I would find it hard to resist, but if there is only a pile of paperwork, I just plow right through and forget to be hungry.

The Reality of Hunger:
Riding Out the Wave

There's no denying that you'll experience hunger during fasting. But it's important to remember that hunger is not as terrible an experience as we expect it to be. We often imagine that hunger will build and build until it is unbearable and we need to stuff ourselves with Krispy Kreme donuts. However, this is not the case at all. The secret is to understand that hunger comes in *waves*. You just need to ride out the waves.

Think back to a time when you skipped lunch. Perhaps you were caught up in a meeting and couldn't get away. At first, you got hungry. The hunger built and built, but there was nothing to be done. But what happened after an hour or so? The hunger entirely dissipated. The wave had passed.

What's the best way to endure the wave of hunger during fasting? Drinking green tea or coffee is often enough. By the time you're finished, the hunger has passed and you've gone on to the next thing to do that day. Hunger is not a continuously growing phenomenon. It will build up, peak, and then dissipate, and all you have to do is ignore it. It will certainly return, but knowing that it will pass once again gives you the power and confidence to handle it.

This even applies to extended fasting periods. Hunger comes quite strongly during the first one or two days of fasting, generally peaking on day two. After that, the hunger just subsides and then goes away. Some people speculate that the ketones generated during fat-burning are actively suppressing appetite. Dr. Ian Gilliland, an expert in endocrinology, wrote about his experiences with fasting patients that "a feeling of well-being is certainly engendered . . . and may amount to euphoria. We did not encounter complaints of hunger after the first day." People weren't hungry and actually felt "euphoric" during fourteen days of fasting. Some people felt so good during fasting that they wanted to continue past the fourteen days. In fact, the absence of hunger during extended fasting is a consistent finding throughout the scientific literature on fasting, as well as in our own IDM Program.

One of the most important things I learned during extended fasting is to be prepared for hunger the first few days by having a list of things to do as a distraction. I kept the list on my refrigerator, and whenever I found myself opening the refrigerator door to look for something to eat, I would stop and choose something off the list to do instead. Distractions included walking, cleaning out a drawer or a cabinet, drinking a glass of water, and anything else I could come up with. It works, and the hunger would be forgotten by the time I was done!

—Kimberly H., Sacramento, CA

I have reversed my insulin resistance with a fasting protocol of 18-hour fasts for 5 days followed by 2 days water-only fasting. I also water-only fast for 10–18 consecutive days every other month. After day 3, all hunger diminishes, ketones soar, and that's when I feel invincible! I feel better at 51 than I ever felt at 21!

**—Debbie F.,
Knoxville, IA**

When people feel they cannot go beyond twenty-four hours of fasting, we sometimes advise them to try three to seven full days of fasting. This sounds completely counterintuitive. If you can't go one day, how can you go seven days? This "hack" works because the extended fasting gives people the chance to experience how hunger can disappear without eating as the body learns how to metabolize its own fat. The long fast rapidly acclimates their bodies to fasting. Once they get over the first one or two days, hunger starts to disappear and they become reassured that they are not overwhelmed by hunger. It is a part of fasting, but not an insurmountable one.

How can people fast for days without being hungry? It comes down to the fact that hunger is not determined by not eating for a certain period of time. Rather, it is a hormonal signal. It does not come about simply because the stomach is empty. When you avoid natural stimuli to hunger, such as the sight and smell of food, as well as the conditioned stimuli to hunger—specific mealtimes, movies, ball games, any event where you normally eat and have learned to expect food—you help avoid that hormonal signal.

Fasting helps to break all the conditioned stimuli and thus helps to *reduce*, not enhance, hunger.

Hunger is a state of mind, not a state of stomach.

References

A. M. Johnstone, P. Faber, E. R. Gibney, M. Elia, G. Horgan, B. E. Golden, and R. J. Stubbs, "Effect of an Acute Fast on Energy Compensation and Feeding Behaviour in Lean Men and Women," *International Journal of Obesity* 26, no. 12 (2002): 1623–28.

Ameneh Madjd, Moira A. Taylor, Alireza Delavari, Reza Malekzadeh, Ian A. Macdonald, and Hamid R. Farshchi, "Effects on Weight Loss in Adults of Replacing Diet Beverages with Water During a Hypoenergetic Diet: A Randomized, 24-wk Clinical Trial," *American Journal of Clinical Nutrition* 102, no. 6: 1305–12. doi: 10.3945/ajcn.115.109397.

I. C. Gilliland, "Total Fasting in the Treatment of Obesity," *Postgraduate Medical Journal* 44, no. 507 (1968): 58–61.

DARRYL

FASTING SUCCESS STORY

Darryl, a sixty-six-year-old man, was referred to me in November 2015 for treatment of his type 2 diabetes, which he'd had for eleven years. He also suffered from high cholesterol and high blood pressure, and he had only one kidney. He had been experiencing significant low back pain, caused in part by his abdominal obesity. Carrying around all that extra weight around his belly threw off his balance and put significant strain on his lower back. Eventually this caused arthritis in his spine and crippling low back pain.

He was referred to a pain specialist, who immediately recognized the classic features of the metabolic syndrome and knew that weight loss would help significantly with his pain.

Darryl's diabetes story was typical. He had started with a small dose of a single medication, but over the years, this had relentlessly increased until he was taking 70 units of insulin daily just to keep his blood sugar under control. We started with a low-carbohydrate, high-fat diet and added some intermittent fasting. He fasted for twenty-four hours at a time three days a week.

The results were immediate. His weight and waist size started decreasing. Within a mere two weeks, we stopped all his insulin because his blood sugars was consistently in the normal range. He has remained off all his diabetic medications since then, and his most recent Hemoglobin A1C measured 5.9 percent, down from 6.8 percent before he started on our program. In other words, despite stopping all his insulin, his blood sugar levels were *better* than ever. In fact, he would not even be classified as a diabetic any longer. His diabetes had completely reversed.

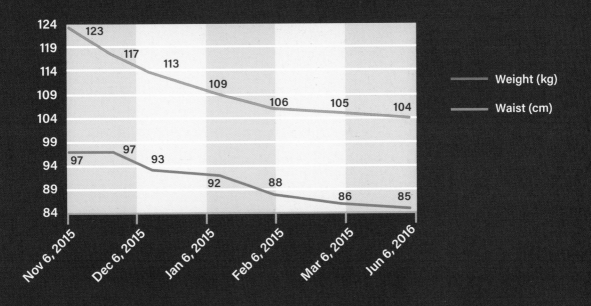

Imagine that. Darryl suffered with type 2 diabetes for eleven years, and at any time, the proper diet could have entirely reversed his diabetes. Darryl could have been injecting himself with insulin for the next twenty years without fixing the underlying problem, but instead, just by following some simple dietary rules, he cured his type 2 diabetes.

Chapter 10
WHO SHOULD NOT FAST?

Now that we've talked about the many benefits of fasting, we need to add a very big caveat: fasting isn't for everyone. It carries certain risks and normal amounts of vitamins, minerals, and other essential nutrients are not ingested. Some people absolutely should not attempt therapeutic fasting, including:

Those who are severely malnourished or underweight

Children under eighteen years of age

Pregnant women

Breastfeeding women

Others should be cautious when fasting but don't necessarily need to avoid it. In the following situations, it is wise to seek the advice of a health-care professional before attempting therapeutic fasting:

You have gout

You are taking medications

You have type 1 or type 2 diabetes

You have gastroesophageal reflux disease

Absolutely Don't Fast If You're:

Severely Malnourished or Underweight

When malnutrition is a concern, it's obviously neither desirable nor wise to deliberately restrict nutrients and calories.

When body fat falls below 4 percent, the body is forced to use protein in order to feed itself. (For comparison, average body fat is 25 percent in men and over 35 percent in women. This is only an average, and an obese person's body fat percentage is far above that. An elite marathoner, despite looking very lean, might have approximately 8 to 10 percent body fat.) The stored energy from fat has run out, and the body must now burn functional tissue to survive. This syndrome is called wasting, and it's neither healthy nor beneficial in any way.

The body mass index (BMI) is calculated by taking your weight in kilograms and dividing it by your height in meters squared: kg/m^2. One well-accepted definition of *underweight* is a BMI of less than 18.5. For a man who stands five-foot-ten, that would correspond to a weight of 129 pounds. I generally advise against any type of fasting at a BMI below 20, as the risk of complications rises dramatically, but it's especially important to avoid longer fasts.

AMY BERGER ▮FASTING ALL-STARS▮

I don't like for people to use fasting as an excuse to eat whatever they want in massive quantities when they're *not* fasting. It should also not be used as a punishment for overeating, "cheating," or "falling off the wagon" of the particular diet program someone is following. It *can* be used as a kind of recalibration or resetting if someone feels they'll benefit from that, but it shouldn't be used as a quick fix to atone for perceived dietary sins.

DOES FASTING CAUSE ANOREXIA?

Patients suffering from anorexia nervosa should clearly not be fasting, since they are already severely underweight and malnourished. Further, fasting may feed directly into the manifestations of anorexia nervosa. Food is the medicine of choice for anorexia, so withholding it is ill-advised. However, does fasting *cause* anorexia?

The simple answer is no. Anorexia is a psychiatric disorder of distorted body image. Patients perceive their bodies as overweight even though they are severely underweight. It is a psychological disease and not one caused by undereating. This is the symptom, not the cause. Fasting is not generally fun, and there is little danger of getting hooked on it. It is certainly not addictive in the way that cocaine is addictive.

Arguing that fasting causes anorexia is like arguing that washing your hands will lead to obsessive-compulsive disorder. Excessive hand-washing is a symptom of the disease, not its cause.

Furthermore, fasting has been practiced safely for thousands of years by millions of people worldwide, but anorexia nervosa is only a very recent phenomenon. If fasting caused anorexia, it would have been described thousands of years ago and affected men as well as women. This argues strongly against fasting as a significant cause. Bottom line? Fasting does not *cause* anorexia—but it should not be attempted by anorexics.

Under Eighteen Years Old

In children, proper growth outweighs all other health concerns, and adequate nutrition is an absolute prerequisite for normal growth. Restricting calories also restricts the essential nutrients necessary for proper growth and the development of vital organs, especially the brain. The normal growth spurt in puberty, in particular, requires tremendous amounts of nutrients. Underfeeding during this period may result in stunted growth, which may be irreversible. In all children under eighteen, the risk of malnutrition during fasting is unacceptably high.

That's not to say that missing a meal here and there is harmful to children's health, but prolonged fasting longer than twenty-four hours is not advisable. This fact has long been recognized by virtually all cultures in the world. Children have always been excluded from cultural or religious fasting to prevent the unintentional development of malnutrition at a critical time of development.

It is more important to teach children about making proper food choices. Choosing to eat whole, unprocessed, natural foods is a good start. Avoiding highly processed grains and especially reducing added sugars also goes a long way toward preventing obesity and promoting good health.

Pregnant

Fasting during pregnancy presents similar concerns about proper fetal development. The developing fetus requires adequate nutrients for optimal growth, and nutrient deficiency may cause irreversible harm during this critical period. For this reason, many women take a specially formulated pregnancy multivitamin. Especially important is folic acid supplementation, as deficiency in folic acid may lead to an increased risk of neural tube defects (for example, the disease spina bifida). Folic acid stores in humans last only several months, so prolonged nutrient deficiency puts the developing fetus at enormous risk.

Since pregnancy is limited to nine months, there is no reason to fast during this time. It may be resumed at a safer time, once the pregnancy (and breastfeeding—see below) is over. Once again, most cultures of the world have long recognized the inherent danger of fasting during this time and exempt pregnant women from cultural and religious fasts.

Breastfeeding

Developing babies receive all their nutrients from the mother in the form of breast milk. If Mom becomes deficient in vitamins and minerals, then the baby will also be deficient. The result may be irreversible growth retardation. For that reason, I do not advise anybody who is breastfeeding to undertake fasting. Missing a meal here or there is certainly not harmful, but deliberate, long-term fasting is not advised.

Again, since breastfeeding is generally limited to months, not years, there is no reason to fast. Once you've finished breastfeeding, you may safely fast without fear of harming your baby.

Fasting is an activity that can be done safely throughout *most* of your adult life, but it is foolish to attempt to fast during those few times when it presents a danger to your own health or the health of your baby. There is simply no reason to rush into it. There is always plenty of time to fast later, when it is safe to do so.

Consult Your Doctor If You:

Have Gout

Gout is an inflammatory arthritis caused by excess uric acid crystals in the joints. High blood levels of uric acid are one of the major contributing factors to this disease, and medications to lower the level of uric acid in the blood are sometimes prescribed to reduce the chance of recurrence.

Uric acid elimination through the urine decreases during fasting, resulting in a rise in uric acid levels. Theoretically, this could worsen gout. In a study of forty-two obese patients who fasted, there was increased uric acid in all patients, but none developed gout.

Most patients with a history of gout tolerate fasting without difficulty. However, knowing the potential risk is important, and if you have any doubts, speak with your physician before starting your fasting regimen.

Are Taking Medications

Anybody who is taking regular medications for any condition *must* consult with their physician before starting any type of dietary or fasting program. Certain medications are best taken with food, which obviously is not possible during fasting. The most common medications that cause problems during fasting are aspirin, metformin, and iron and magnesium supplements. But it is often possible to arrange the fasting schedule to accommodate these medications.

Aspirin is commonly used as a blood-thinner in people with cardiovascular disease. One common side effect is gastritis—the irritation of the lining of the stomach. In severe cases, it may cause ulcers to form in the stomach and small intestine. Aspirin is often taken with food to lessen the risk of these complications. Many aspirin tablets are now coated with a protective film to protect the lining of the stomach, but the risk of gastritis and ulcers is only reduced, not eliminated. Taking aspirin without food raises the risk of stomach irritation.

Metformin is the most widely prescribed medication in the world for type 2 diabetes. This blood-sugar-lowering medication has been used since the 1950s and is also commonly prescribed for polycystic ovary syndrome. One major side effect is gastrointestinal upset, which may become worse on an empty stomach. The most commonly reported symptoms are diarrhea and nausea or vomiting.

Iron supplement tablets are commonly prescribed for low blood counts due to chronic blood loss, also called iron deficiency anemia. For example, many women have heavy monthly periods that lead to low iron levels. Among the most common side effects of iron supplements are both constipation and abdominal pain, which may be made worse by fasting.

Magnesium is a mineral stored largely in the bones. Supplements are often taken to treat leg cramps, migraine headaches, and restless leg syndrome. It is also used as an antacid and laxative. Magnesium supplements taken orally are often poorly absorbed through the intestines, leading to diarrhea. Taking magnesium with food often reduces these symptoms. Low magnesium levels are particularly common in type 2 diabetes.

As an alternative, magnesium may be absorbed through the skin through Epsom salts, crystals of magnesium sulphate. You can dissolve a full cup of Epsom salts in a tub of warm water and soak for thirty minutes. The magnesium will be absorbed through the skin. This is a traditional remedy for many things, including muscle cramps, constipation, and skin problems. Alternatively, there are preparations of magnesium oil or magnesium gel that may be applied to the skin.

Have Diabetes

If you have type 1 or type 2 diabetes, it's essential to be particularly careful while fasting or even just changing dietary patterns. This is especially true if you are taking medications. If you continue the same dose of medication but reduce food intake, there is a risk of your blood sugar going extremely low—a situation called hypoglycemia.

Symptoms of hypoglycemia include shaking, sweating, irritability or nervousness, feeling faint, hunger, and nausea. More severe symptoms include confusion, delirium, and seizures. Untreated, hypoglycemia may even lead to death. Symptoms may appear very rapidly, and if they do, you must quickly ingest some sugary beverage or food to reverse this life-threatening situation.

You *must* consult with a physician to adjust the doses of diabetic medications or insulin before starting any dietary program. Careful monitoring of blood sugars is crucially important. If you cannot do this, then you should not attempt fasting. (See page 140 for more on fasting with diabetes.)

Have Gastroesophageal Reflux Disease

In gastroesophageal reflux disease (GERD), commonly known as heartburn, stomach acid backs up into the esophagus, causing damage to the sensitive tissues of the esophagus. This feels like a dull pain in the lower chest or upper abdomen and often becomes worse when lying down. People often describe feeling their stomach contents "coming back up."

Excessive abdominal fat places increased pressure on the stomach and forces food and stomach acid back up into the esophagus. This can occasionally be made worse during fasting because there is nothing in the stomach to absorb the stomach acid. (This is mildly, and sadly, ironic, since fasting is often undertaken for the purpose of losing weight, which should ultimately make the heartburn better.) After weight loss is achieved, heartburn often resolves. Sometimes fasting improves symptoms of heartburn because food can stimulate the production of stomach acid, so fasting reduces it.

Here are some simple techniques to help reduce symptoms of GERD:

- Avoid foods that aggravate reflux—including chocolate, caffeine, alcohol, fried foods, and citrus. Caffeine relaxes the lower esophageal sphincter, which may worsen reflux.
- Finish eating at least three hours before bed.
- Go for a walk after dinner.
- Elevate the head of the bed with blocks.
- Try alkaline water or water with lemon.
- Take over-the-counter medications such as antacids, bismuth solutions, or ranitidine (Zantac).
- Ask your physician about stronger prescription medications, such as proton pump inhibitors.

If these strategies do not work, it is often possible to modify the fasting regimen to avoid heartburn. For example, rather than doing a true fast, try eating a handful of salad greens at regular intervals. This preserves most of the benefits of the fast while alleviating the symptoms of heartburn. A "fat fast," in which only fat is eaten during the fasting period, may also be effective—see page 194.

Should Women Fast?

I'm often asked whether women should fast. I am not sure where the rumor that women *shouldn't* fast started, but I have heard it often enough to address this question specifically.

There is some persistent concern that women may not experience the same benefits of fasting as men. Nothing could be further from the truth. Virtually all studies on fasting confirm that both men and women benefit from fasting. Further, there is no particular difference in efficacy between the two sexes.

My own clinical experience confirms this. Having helped hundreds of men and women fast over the last five years, I've seen no difference between the sexes. If anything, women tend to do better. Many of our greatest success stories are women. Megan, program director, improved her health so much with fasting protocols that she left her career in medical research to help others succeed with fasting. While women can, of course, have

Men

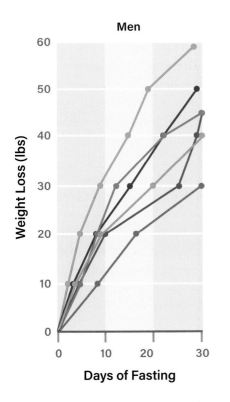

Women

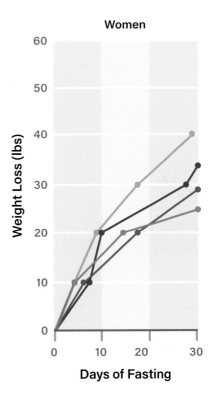

Source: Drenick, Hunt, and Swendseid, "Influence of Fasting and Refeeding on Body Composition."

Figure 10.1. Men and women have similar rates of weight loss during fasting.

problems during fasting, men often have the same troubles, too. Interestingly, I've seen the highest success rates with husbands and wives who try fasting together: the mutual support is a big help and makes fasting far easier.

Fasting has been part of human culture for at least two thousand years. Are Muslim women exempt from fasting? Are Buddhist women exempt from fasting? Are Catholic women exempt from fasting? Nope! With thousands of years of practical fasting experience, none of these religions make a distinction between adult men and women, except when women are pregnant or breastfeeding.

One area of specific concern with women is that fasting could affect reproductive hormones. Certainly, malnourished women should not fast, since excessively low body fat can lead to amenorrhea (loss of menstrual cycles) and difficulty conceiving. But normal-weight women do not see a significant difference in their sex hormone profile during fasting. One study examined the effect of a three-day fast on the reproductive hormones during different parts of the menstrual cycle. Glucose and insulin levels stayed low, showing compliance with the fast, but all reproductive hormones remained within normal limits. Ultrasound also demonstrated normal growth of the dominant follicle (egg), and menstrual cycles remained unchanged. The problems of amenorrhea and anovulatory cycles (menstrual cycles where no egg is produced) arise when body fat percentage falls too low. However, women with excessively low body fat should not be

DR. MICHAEL RUSCIO ▪ FASTING ALL-STARS

It's important to track whatever your key symptoms are. It's also important to assess if globally you appear to be getting better or worse as the days go on. If you are generally getting better, then stick with it.

If you feel you are generally getting worse, then your current approach may not be suited for you and you might want to try a different fasting approach.

fasting in the first place (neither should men, for that matter). If amenorrhea or any other menstrual problems appear during fasting, stop immediately.

Pregnant and breastfeeding women, as previously noted, should not fast. These are situations that absolutely require adequate nutrients for growth.

Let's be clear. There are certainly potential problems women may face during fasting. But all these problems come up with men, too. Sometimes women don't lose weight the way they want—and sometimes neither do men. Sometimes women find that fasting is difficult—as do men. The studies on fasting, many going back over a hundred years, all show that it's safe for both sexes.

The most important thing to always remember is that if you are feeling poorly in *any way*, whether you are a man or a woman, you must stop fasting immediately and contact your health-care provider.

References

D. A. Johnston and K. G. Wormsley, "The Effects of Fasting on 24-h Gastric Secretion of Patients with Duodenal Ulcers Resistant to Ranitidine," *Alimentary Pharmacology and Therapeutics* 3, no. 5 (1989): 471–9, doi: 10.1111/j.1365-2036.1989.tb00238.x.

E. J. Drenick, I. F. Hunt, and M. E. Swendseid, "Influence of Fasting and Refeeding on Body Composition," *American Journal of Public Health* 58, no. 3 (1968): 477–84.

I. C. Gilliland, "Total Fasting in the Treatment of Obesity," *Postgraduate Medical Journal* 44, no. 507 (1968): 58–61.

J. Runcie and T. J. Thomson, "Total Fasting, Hyperuricaemia and Gout," *Postgraduate Medical Journal* 45, no. 522 (1969): 251–3.

Kristin K. Hoddy, Cynthia M. Kroeger, John F. Trepanowski, Adrienne R. Barnosky, Surabhi Bhutani, and Krista K. Varady, "Safety of Alternate Day Fasting and Effect on Disordered Eating Behaviors," *Nutrition Journal* 14, no. 44 (2015), doi: 10.1186/s12937-015-0029-9.

M. R. Soules, M. C. Merriggiola, R. A. Steiner, D. K. Clifton, B. Toivola, and W. J. Bremner, "Short-Term Fasting in Normal Women: Absence of Effects on Gonadotrophin Secretion and the Menstrual Cycle," *Clinical Endocrinology* 40, no. 6 (1994): 725–31.

Part Two

HOW TO FAST

Chapter 11
KINDS OF FASTS AND BEST PRACTICES

It's useful to categorize fasts by two features: what is allowed on the fast and how long or frequent the fast is. We'll take up the questions of length and frequency in Chapters 12, 13, and 14, but first, let's look at the different kinds of fasts in terms of what may be consumed.

Most definitions of fasting allow noncaloric drinks only. This means that water, tea, and black coffee are all allowed during fasting, but sugar, honey, fructose, agave nectar, and other sugars are prohibited. There is some disagreement about artificial sweeteners like stevia, aspartame, and sucralose. Since there are no calories in these, technically, they could be allowed. However, the use of chemicals in these artificial sweeteners defeats the spirit of fasting, which is to cleanse or purify the body, not only from unwanted sugars and fats but also from chemicals and other artificial agents. The same argument applies to artificial flavors, such as those in Crystal Light or Kool-Aid, and to bouillon cubes.

The water-only fast is a traditional and classic variant—all other beverages and additives are not permitted during the fasting period. It's important to note that this fast generally includes zero salt. Without salt, the body cannot hold onto water, and therefore there is some risk of dehydration. Some variants of the water-only fast allow you to drink salt water, although it can be difficult to get down. However, the body has a remarkable ability to retain salt when it is not readily available in the diet. This means that as long as the water-only fast is limited in duration, your salt requirements will be fairly low, and salt deficiency shouldn't be a problem.

Juice fasting permits the consumption of juice as well as water. Since juices naturally contain sugars and calories, this is not technically a true fast, but the word is often used in this context. Results of this fast will vary depending upon the type and amount of juice consumed. Fruit juices tend to be very high in sugar and therefore will often not produce as good a result as other, stricter fasts. "Green" juice fasting has recently surged in popularity. As you might guess from the name, this involves juicing green leafy vegetables, like spinach and kale. The resulting juice contains far less sugar than the juice of sweet fruits like oranges and apples. In addition, leafy vegetables contain little actual juice, so the leaves are often ground up and blended with the juice, which provides fiber and nutrients. Celery is often juiced in this mixture, too.

The "fat fast" is a newer variation of fasting. Relatively pure fats, such as coconut oil, cream, and butter, are allowed during this fast, so it, too, is not a true fast. Fat is normally not eaten in isolation—we rarely drink a cup of olive oil or eat a pat of butter by itself—but some people feel that eating fat this way helps reduce hunger and makes fasting much easier.

The popularity of "bulletproof coffee" has helped this trend. To make coffee "bulletproof," you add fat in the form of coconut

AMY BERGER ▐ FASTING ALL-STARS

During a fast, small amounts of pure fat or almost pure fat (a spoonful of olive or coconut oil, a pat of butter), and for some, even a very small amount of solid food, such as macadamia nuts or walnuts— something that is primarily fat with a negligible amount of carbohydrate and little to no protein—can be consumed without interfering with the physiological benefits of the fast. Sometimes just having a small bite of something like this can help a person stick to a fast when they might otherwise be struggling, and these foods are unlikely to be obstacles to getting the desired results.

oil, medium-chain triglycerides (MCT oil), or butter from grass-fed cows. The high fat content of the coffee gives this drink a substantial number of calories (400 to 500 per cup, depending upon the recipe), so this would be more accurately termed a meal replacement. However, virtually all of the calories are derived from fat. (See page 264 for a recipe for Bulletproof Coffee.)

There are a number of purported benefits to the fat fast. Some claim that it helps weight loss as part of a ketogenic or very low carbohydrate diet, in which the body burns fat for energy. Others feel that the fat helps with mental clarity or that it helps kill cravings. While scientific proof of the effectiveness of the fat fast is currently scarce, anecdotes of success abound.

In a "dry fast," no fluids of any kind are allowed. Muslims practice this type of fasting during the daylight hours of the holy month of Ramadan. This combines fasting with mild dehydration. In my opinion, this makes fasting much more difficult than other types of fast, and I do not recommend this for medical reasons. The risk of complications is also much higher due to the accompanying dehydration.

The "fasting-mimicking diet" is a diet created by researchers to re-create the benefits of fasting without actual fasting. It is a complicated regimen of reduced caloric intake over five days every month. The first day allows 1,090 calories, composed of 10 percent protein, 56 percent fat, and 34 percent carbohydrate. That's

FASTING ALL-STARS DR. THOMAS SEYFRIED

All types of fasts can have therapeutic benefit. The key to therapy is prolonged therapeutic ketosis (blood ketones in the range of 3–6mM), together with reduced blood glucose levels (3–4 mM). Patients will need to use the Precision Xtra meter from Abbott to determine when they can enter the therapeutic zone. GKI ratios of 1.0 or below would best represent the therapeutic range.

followed by four days of 725 calories, with the same nutritional breakdown. There is sparse data to support the claim that this diet provides all the benefits of fasting, and I don't recommend it because of its unnecessary complexity. To me, it is far simpler to follow five days of regular fasting per month.

Intensive Dietary Management Fasting: Best Practices

We use fasting extensively in the Intensive Dietary Management (IDM) Program for weight loss and other metabolic disorders, such as type 2 diabetes and fatty liver disease. Regardless of the duration of your fast, the general guidelines outlined here will help you fast in a healthy way. Certain aspects may work for you; others may not. You are always free to experiment and adjust, as there are no hard and fast rules.

The IDM fast permits water, tea, and coffee. Sugar, honey, agave nectar, and other sweeteners are not permitted. Artificial sweeteners or flavors are not allowed, but natural flavors such as lemon juice, mint, cinnamon, or other spices are.

The IDM fast also allows homemade bone broth, which both makes fasting easier and may help prevent salt deficiency during longer fasts.

Water

Be sure to stay well hydrated throughout your fast. Water, both still and sparkling, is always a good choice. Aim to drink two liters of water and other fluids daily. As a good practice, start every day with eight ounces of cool water to ensure adequate hydration. Add a squeeze of lemon or lime to flavor the water, if you wish. Alternatively, you can add orange slices, berries, or cucumber slices to a pitcher of water for an infusion of flavor. Diluted apple-cider vinegar in water may help lower your blood sugar. However, artificial flavors and sweeteners are prohibited. Kool-Aid, Crystal Light, or Tang should *not* be added to your water.

I've lost over 50 pounds (went from 215 to 165) and maintained it. As a matter of routine, I eat LCHF and intermittent fast for a minimum of 18 hours, and I do a water-only fast for 2 to 3 days a week. I can't say I enjoy the water-only fasts, but there's no denying that they've helped me break through weight-loss plateaus. I find keeping busy is the best way to get through a water-only fast.

—Philip M., Bellaire, TX

Tea

All types of tea are excellent choices, including green, black, oolong, and herbal. Green tea is an especially good choice during a fast: the catechins in green tea are believed to help suppress appetite. Teas can be blended together for variety and can be enjoyed hot or cold. Spices such as cinnamon or nutmeg add flavor.

Herbal teas are not true teas because they do not contain tea leaves. However, they also are great for fasting. Cinnamon tea and ginger tea have both been used for their reputed appetite-suppressing power. Mint tea and chamomile tea are often used for their soothing properties. Because herbal teas contain no caffeine, they can be enjoyed anytime during the day or night. All teas, including herbal teas, can be enjoyed either hot or cold.

Adding a small amount of cream or milk to your tea is acceptable (see below), but sugar and artificial sweeteners and flavors are not allowed. However, if you are finding progress slow, you may want to eliminate all calories completely during fasting. We often advise patients to go back to a classic water-only fast if they hit a stubborn weight plateau.

Coffee

Coffee, both caffeinated and decaffeinated, is permitted during a fast. We also permit a small amount of cream or coconut oil to be added to coffee or tea. While this does technically mean it's not a true fast, the effect is small enough that it seems to make no difference to the overall outcome of the fast. Furthermore, this flexibility may improve your ability to stick to the program. By "small amount," we mean 1 to 2 teaspoons of cream or coconut oil—nowhere near the copious amounts of fat used in bulletproof coffee.

Spices such as cinnamon or nutmeg may also be added, but not sweeteners, sugar, or artificial flavors. On hot days, iced coffee is a great alternative. Simply brew a pot as you normally would and let it cool in the refrigerator. Coffee has many health benefits that are just being recognized—for instance, it may reduce the risk of type 2 diabetes and is a great source of antioxidants.

Bone Broth

Homemade bone broth, made from beef, pork, chicken, or fish bones, is a good choice for fasting days. Animal bones are simmered with other vegetables and seasonings for long periods of time, anywhere from eight to thirty-six hours—see page 266 for a recipe. Vegetable broth is a suitable alternative, although bone broth contains more nutrients. All vegetables, herbs, and spices are great additions to bone broth, but do not add bouillon cubes, which are full of artificial flavors and monosodium glutamate. Beware of canned broths: they are poor imitations of the homemade kind.

We often advise people to add a good pinch of sea salt to their homemade bone broth. During longer fasts, it is possible to become deficient in salt since it is not taken with water, tea, or coffee, and salt deficiency can lead to dehydration. Sea salt also contains other trace minerals, such as potassium and magnesium, which may be particularly beneficial during fasting. (For shorter fasts, such as the twenty-four- and thirty-six-hour variety, it probably makes little difference.)

There is also a small amount of protein and some minerals (calcium and magnesium) in bone broth, so technically, any fast that allows broth is not a true fast. But many people have found that the broth makes a longer-duration fast much more bearable. The gelatin and protein contained in the broth help diminish hunger pangs, and there are numerous other health benefits ascribed to bone broth, including anti-inflammatory effects and benefits for bone and joint health.

Chapter 12
INTERMITTENT FASTING

In Part I, I've argued that fasting isn't bad for you—in fact, it was a regular part of human society for thousands of years, and there are benefits to it for those who are dealing with certain health issues—in particular, obesity and type 2 diabetes—in today's world of constant food abundance.

Traditional hunter-gatherer societies virtually never develop obesity or diabetes, even during times of plentiful food. In the pre-agricultural era, it is estimated that animal foods provided about two-thirds of the calories in the human diet. So, despite all the modern teeth gnashing about red meat and saturated fats, it seems that our ancestors had little problems eating them.

About ten thousand years ago, with the agricultural revolution and its greater reliability of food, we developed the habit of eating two or three times per day. But many early agricultural societies ate carbohydrate-based diets without problems with obesity. It seems to be a modern problem.

From these historical examples, we can see that it is certainly possible to eat meat and carbohydrates without the problem of diabesity in a society. What matters most is our insulin response to food, since obesity is largely a problem of excessive insulin. And when it comes to insulin, as we've discussed in Chapters 5 and 6, the timing and frequency of meals is as important as the composition of the meal. That is, the question of *when* to eat is as important as *what* to eat. It is precisely here that intermittent fasting may help us the most.

What Is Intermittent Fasting?

The term *intermittent fasting* simply means that periods of fasting occur regularly between periods of normal eating. How long each period of fasting lasts, and how long the period of normal eating lasts, can vary widely. There are many different fasting regimens, and there's no "best" one. They all work to different degrees for different people. One regimen may work for one person but be utterly ineffective for the next. One person may prefer shorter fasts while another prefers longer ones. Neither is correct or incorrect. It is all personal preference.

Fasts can range from twelve hours to three months or more. You can fast once a week or once a month or once a year. Shorter fasts are generally done more frequently, even daily, while longer fasts—twenty-four to thirty-six hours is the most common duration—are usually done two to three times per week. Prolonged fasting may range from one week to one month.

I categorize fasting periods as short (less than twenty-four hours) or long (more than twenty-four hours), but this is somewhat arbitrary. In the IDM Program, shorter regimens are generally used by those mostly interested in weight loss rather than in treating type 2 diabetes, fatty liver disease, or other metabolic diseases. However, shorter, more frequent fasts still often work well for these conditions.

During short-duration fasts, you are still eating daily, which minimizes the risk of malnutrition. Shorter fasts also fit into work and family-life schedules easily.

AMY BERGER ■ FASTING ALL-STARS

I think intermittent fasting is great. Done on a regular basis, the body gets accustomed to it and you don't think twice about it. Your hunger signals will become more regular—that is, they'll adjust to the fasting and you'll start to become hungry when your body is ready to eat, rather than from "false" signals being driven by wild fluctuations in insulin, blood glucose, and stress hormones.

Longer-duration fasts give quicker results but are usually done less frequently. Fasting for more than twenty-four hours may sound difficult, but I've found that a surprising number of patients prefer to fast longer and less frequently. We'll look at longer fasts in Chapters 13 and 14.

Remember, you can always switch from one fasting regimen to the other. You are never locked in. But keep in mind that the first several fasting periods are always difficult, and unfortunately there is not much you can do about that. Like everything else in life, fasting becomes easier the more you do it.

Short Daily Fasting Regimens

12-Hour Fasts

In years past, a daily twelve-hour fasting period was considered a normal eating pattern. You would eat three meals a day from, say, 7 a.m. to 7 p.m., and then fast from 7 p.m. to 7 a.m. At that point, you would "break your fast" with a small breakfast. This was pretty standard until the 1970s, and perhaps not coincidentally, there also was much less obesity back then.

Two major dietary changes happened starting in 1977. With the publication of the USDA's *Dietary Guidelines for Americans* that year, we changed to a higher-carbohydrate, lower-fat diet. Diets high in refined carbohydrates stimulate constant, high levels of insulin, which makes people gain weight and, eventually, become obese.

FASTING ALL-STARS DR. BERT HERRING

A fasting schedule cannot correct appetite permanently; the correction is effective only when the fasting schedule is maintained, though a day or two off schedule does not immediately erase the appetite correction effect.

Figure 12.1. Insulin levels during a traditional 12-hour fasting schedule with three meals a day.

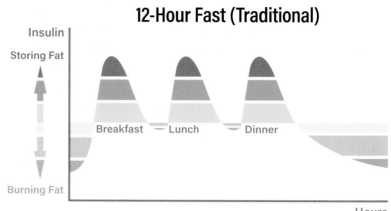

12-Hour Fast (Traditional)

Insulin

Storing Fat

Breakfast   Lunch   Dinner

Burning Fat

Hours

Figure 12.2. Insulin levels during a 16-hour fasting schedule with an 8-hour eating window. You could easily eat three times within that window rather than twice, as the graph shows.

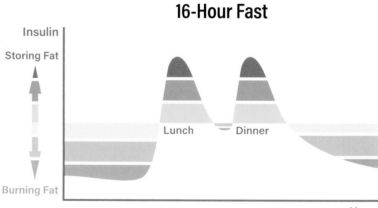

16-Hour Fast

Insulin

Storing Fat

Lunch   Dinner

Burning Fat

Hours

Figure 12.3. Insulin levels during a 20-hour fasting schedule, with all meals eaten within a four-hour window in the evening.

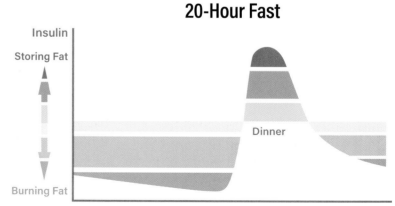

20-Hour Fast

Insulin

Storing Fat

Dinner

Burning Fat

Hours

The other critical, though rarely recognized, dietary change was the gradual increase in meal frequency. In 1977, eating opportunities (both meals and snacks) averaged three per day—breakfast, lunch, and dinner. By 2003, that figure was closer to six per day. People were eating three meals and three snacks daily, and insulin levels were beginning to be kept perpetually high. Over time, the constant stimulation of insulin leads to the development of insulin resistance, which leads back to high insulin levels, which, in turn, leads to obesity. (See Chapters 5 and 6 for more on insulin and insulin resistance.)

Daily twelve-hour fasting introduces a period of very low insulin levels during the day. This prevents the development of insulin resistance, making the twelve-hour fast a powerful preventative weapon against obesity. In fact, the combination of whole foods, lower-carbohydrate diets, less added sugars, and a daily twelve-hour fast was enough to prevent most Americans in the 1950s and 1960s from developing obesity—even though they still ate plenty of white bread and jam, and whole-wheat bread was rare and whole-wheat pasta unheard-of.

But while a daily twelve-hour fast may be a great preventative strategy, it may not be powerful enough to *reverse* weight gain. Slightly longer fasting periods are often required for that.

16-Hour Fasts

This regimen incorporates a sixteen-hour period of fasting into your daily meal schedule. For example, you might fast from 7 p.m. to 11 a.m. daily. You could also say that you have an eight-hour eating window every day. For that reason, it is sometimes called

FASTING ALL-STARS ABEL JAMES

For most people, I recommend 16:8 intermittent fasting (a compressed eating window) over longer-term fasting. The fact that you sleep through the majority of your fast makes it relatively painless.

time-restricted eating. On this schedule, most people skip the morning meal every day. But how many meals you eat within that eight-hour window is your choice. Some people choose to eat two meals during that window and others eat three.

A Swedish bodybuilder named Martin Berkhan popularized this regimen, which is sometimes called the LeanGains method. Several years afterwards, a book called *The 8-Hour Diet* espoused the same eight-hour eating window.

A major advantage of the sixteen-hour fast is that it is fairly simple to incorporate into everyday life. For most people, it only means skipping breakfast and eating lunch and dinner within eight hours of each other. Many people do not feel hungry in the morning despite skipping breakfast and find this method extremely easy to implement.

The daily sixteen-hour fast certainly has more power than the daily twelve-hour fast, but it should be combined with a low-carbohydrate diet for the best effect. Weight loss on this regimen tends to be slow and steady.

20-Hour Fasts: "The Warrior Diet"

In his 2002 book *The Warrior Diet*, Ori Hofmekler stresses that the timing of meals matters almost as much as their composition—as I discussed earlier, both the "when to eat" and "what to eat" questions are important, but "when" is seriously underappreciated.

Hofmekler, drawing upon inspiration from ancient warrior tribes such as the Spartans and Romans, devised a "warrior diet" in which all meals are eaten in the evening during a four-hour window. This results in a twenty-hour fasting period each day. Hofmekler's diet also emphasizes natural, unprocessed foods and high-intensity interval training, both of which I believe to be healthy practices.

Circadian Rhythms

Circadian rhythms are repetitive, predictable, cyclical changes in behaviors and hormones over twenty-four hours. These patterns are seen in most animals. Almost all our hormones, including growth hormone, cortisol, and parathyroid hormone, are secreted in a circadian rhythm. Circadian rhythms also help govern insulin, which affects weight gain, and ghrelin, which controls hunger— leading to practical implications for eating patterns and weight loss.

Insulin and Nighttime Eating

Circadian rhythms have evolved to respond to differences predominantly in ambient light, as determined by the season and time of day. It is believed that food was relatively scarce in Paleolithic times and was predominantly available during daylight hours. Humans hunted and ate by day, and once the sun went down, well, you just couldn't see the food in front of your face. Nocturnal animals may very well have circadian rhythms more suited to eating at night, but not humans.

Given that, is there a difference between eating during the day and eating at night? Well, the studies are few, but perhaps revealing. In a 2013 study, two groups of overweight women were randomly assigned to eat a large breakfast or a large dinner. Both ate 1400 calories per day; only the timing of the largest meal was changed.

The breakfast group lost far more weight than the dinner group. Why? Despite following similar diets and eating about the same amount, the dinner group had a much larger overall rise in insulin. An earlier 1992 study showed similar results. In response to the

FASTING ALL-STARS ROBB WOLF

If you're in a high-stress environment, IF may be a bit too much to deal with. Hard-training athletes need to be careful in how they roll out an IF protocol. There is some indication IF can enhance fat adaptation (particularly when in concert with a nutritional ketosis protocol), but I have also seen folks get into "deep water" by chronically undereating. Fasting is a powerful tool, but like all tools, you really need to consider why you are using it and what the specific context is.

same meal given either early or late in the day, the insulin response was 25 to 50 percent greater in the evening.

Weight gain is driven by insulin, and the higher insulin response in the evening was translating into more weight gain for the dinner group. This illustrates the very important point that obesity is a hormonal, not a caloric, imbalance, and it may help explain the well-known association of night shift work and obesity. (However, that could also have to do with the increased cortisol response due to disturbed sleep.)

Eating the largest meal in the evening seems to cause a much larger rise in insulin than eating earlier. Folk wisdom, of course, also advises to avoid eating large meals in the evening. The reason offered usually is something along the lines of, "If you eat just before bed, you don't get a chance to burn it off and it will turn to fat." Maybe that's not technically true, but perhaps there is something here. Eating late at night seems to be especially problematic for weight gain. This response may have evolved to *help* us gain fat, which may have had a survival advantage in times past.

Ghrelin and Hunger Patterns

Hunger, too, has a natural circadian rhythm. If hunger were simply due to lack of food, we would consistently be hungry in the morning after the long overnight fast. But personal experience and studies show that hunger is *lowest* in the morning, and breakfast is typically the smallest, not the largest, meal of the day. Hunger follows a natural, circadian rhythm that is independent of the eat/fast cycle.

Ghrelin, the hunger hormone, rises and falls in a natural circadian rhythm, with a low at 8:00 a.m. and a high at 8:00 p.m. Correspondingly, hunger typically falls to its lowest level at 7:50 a.m. and peaks at 7:50 p.m. These are natural rhythms inherent in our genetic makeup. Hunger is not so simple as "the longer you don't eat, the hungrier you'll be." Hormonal regulation of hunger plays a key role.

Interestingly, during extended fasting, ghrelin peaks during the first two days and then steadily falls. This aligns perfectly with what we see clinically: hunger is the worst problem on the first two days, but many people on longer fasts report that hunger typically disappears after day 2.

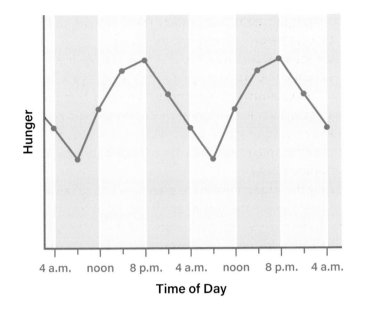

Figure 12.4. Due to circadian rhythms, hunger is naturally lowest at 8:00 a.m. and highest at 8:00 p.m.

Source: Scheer, Morris, and Shea, "The Internal Circadian Clock Increases Hunger and Appetite in the Evening Independent of Food Intake and Other Behaviors."

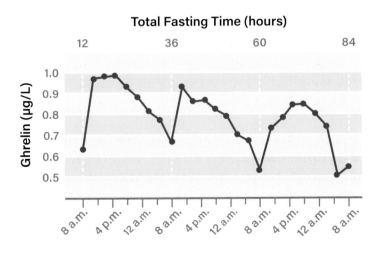

Figure 12.5. Ghrelin, the hormone that regulates hunger, peaks on day 2 during a prolonged fast.

Source: Espelund et al., "Fasting Unmasks a Strong Inverse Association Between Ghrelin and Cortisol in Serum: Studies in Obese and Normal-Weight Subjects."

Timing the Largest Meal of the Day

So, what's the practical implication of these hormonal rhythms for daily eating?

At 8 a.m., our hunger is actively suppressed. It is counterproductive to force-feed ourselves then. What's the point? Eating does not produce weight loss. Forcing ourselves to eat at a time when we are not hungry is not a winning strategy.

Eating late at night is also a poor strategy. Hunger is maximally stimulated at approximately 7:50 p.m. At this time, insulin is maximally stimulated by food, which means that the same amount of food results in higher insulin levels. This higher insulin level will naturally drive weight gain.

Unfortunately, that timing coincides with the largest meal of the day in North America. Making dinner the biggest meal of the day is mostly driven not by health concerns but by the hours of the workday and school. Shift workers are at a particular disadvantage. They tend to eat larger meals even later in the evening, leading to higher insulin.

So the optimal strategy seems to be eating the largest meal in the midday, sometime between noon and 3:00 p.m., and only a small amount in the evening hours. Interestingly, this is the traditional Mediterranean eating pattern. They eat a large lunch, followed by a siesta in the afternoon, and then have a small, almost snack-sized dinner. While we often think of the Mediterranean diet as healthy due to the type of foods in it, the timing of meals in the Mediterranean may also play a role.

References

Daniela Jakubowicz, Maayan Barnea, Julio Wainstein, and Oren Froy, "High Caloric Intake at Breakfast vs. Dinner Differentially Influences Weight Loss of Overweight and Obese Women," *Obesity* 21 (2013): 2504–21.

E. Van Cauter, E. T. Shapiro, H. Tillil, and K. S. Polonsky, "Circadian Modulation of Glucose and Insulin Responses to Meals: Relationship to Cortisol Rhythm," *American Journal of Physiology: Endocrinology and Metabolism* 262, no. 4 (1992): E467–E475.

F. A. Scheer, C. J. Morris, and S. A. Shea, "The Internal Circadian Clock Increases Hunger and Appetite in the Evening Independent of Food Intake and Other Behaviors," *Obesity* 21, no. 3 (2013): 421–3.

L. Cordain, S. B. Eaton, J. Brand Miller, N. Mann, and K. Hill, "The Paradoxical Nature of Hunter-Gatherer Diets: Meat-Based, yet Non-Atherogenic," *European Journal of Clinical Nutrition* 56, suppl. 1 (2002): S42–S52.

Satchidananda Panda, John B. Hogenesch, and Steve A. Kay, "Circadian Rhythms from Flies to Human," *Nature* 417, no. 6886 (2002): 329–35, doi: 10.1038/417329a.

U. Espelund, T. K. Hansen, K. Hollund, H. Beck-Nielsen, J. T. Clausen, B. S. Hansen, H. Orskoy, J. O. Jorgensen, and J. Frystyk, "Fasting Unmasks a Strong Inverse Association Between Ghrelin and Cortisol in Serum: Studies in Obese and Normal-Weight Subjects," *Journal of Clinical Endocrinology and Metabolism* 90, no. 2 (2005): 741–6.

Chapter 13
LONGER PERIODS OF FASTING

In Part I, we talked about how insulin and insulin resistance are at the heart of both obesity and type 2 diabetes. Since all foods increase insulin to some degree, the most efficient method of lowering insulin is eating nothing at all. Even shorter fasts of less than twenty-four hours can prevent the development of insulin resistance and reverse relatively minor levels of resistance, and they certainly help with weight loss.

But because breaking insulin resistance requires not just low insulin levels but *persistently low* levels, we need longer fasting periods.

The Risks and Benefits of Longer Fasts

During longer-duration fasts, health benefits—including weight loss and reduced insulin levels—accrue quickly, but there is also a higher risk of complications for diabetics and those who are taking medications. I've found longer fasts to be particularly helpful in treating type 2 diabetics and recalcitrant obesity cases because they are more powerful than shorter fasts. However, I always monitor patients' blood pressure, vital signs, and blood work very closely. I cannot stress enough that *if you do not feel well at any point, you must stop fasting.* You can be hungry, but you should not feel sick.

If you are on medication, you must be carefully monitored by a physician during fasting—and of course, make sure to talk to your doctor before beginning a fasting regimen or making changes to your diet. This is particularly important if you're on diabetes medications. During longer fasts, the reduced intake of food often lowers blood glucose. If you take the same dose of medication as you would on a normal eating day, there is a high risk of becoming hypoglycemic, which is very dangerous.

Symptoms of hypoglycemia include confusion, sweating, and tremors. You may also experience a feeling of hunger, shakiness, or weakness. Left untreated, it may advance to loss of consciousness, seizures, and, in extreme cases, death.

Lower blood sugar is not a complication per se, because it's expected during fasting. We *want* to lower blood sugar. But it does mean that if you're taking medication to lower your blood sugar, you are overmedicated when you're fasting. Blood sugar and medications must be carefully matched in order to avoid both low and high blood sugar. You must work very carefully with a physician to adjust medications and monitor blood sugar on a fasting regimen.

In general, diabetic medications and insulin *must* be reduced on the fasting day to avoid hypoglycemia. Exactly how much to reduce it should be overseen by your physician.

Make sure that if you're taking medication, you talk to your physician before trying a longer fast!

24-Hour Fasts

A twenty-four-hour fast involves fasting from dinner to dinner, or breakfast to breakfast, whatever you prefer. For example, if you finish dinner at 7 p.m. on day 1, you would then fast until having dinner at 7 p.m. on day 2. Despite the name, you do not actually go a full day without eating, since you are still taking one meal on the fasting day. In essence, you are eating a single meal for that day.

This fasting regimen has several important advantages compared to other longer fasts. Because you still eat a meal on the fasting day, you can take any medications that must be taken with food, such as metformin, iron supplements, or aspirin.

This fasting regimen is also the most easily incorporated into everyday life. You can fast without disrupting family dinners—it really only involves skipping breakfast and lunch. It's particularly easy during a busy day at work. You start the morning with a large cup of coffee, skipping breakfast, then work right through lunch and get home in time for dinner. This saves both time and money. There is no cleanup or cooking for breakfast. You'll be home for dinner without anybody even realizing you were fasting.

Nutrient deficiency is not a major concern with a twenty-four-hour fast. Since you are still eating daily, you just need to make sure that during that meal you consume adequate proteins, vitamins, and minerals by eating nutrient-dense, natural, unprocessed foods. You could follow this regimen daily, although most will get good results doing a twenty-four-hour fast two to three times per week. Brad Pilon, the author of *Eat, Stop, Eat*, recommends using a twenty-four-hour fast twice a week.

EATING AROUND A LONGER FAST

When you're following a regular fasting regimen that involves longer fasts, it's best not to deliberately restrict calories after your fast. You should still remain on a low-carbohydrate, high-fat, unprocessed-food diet, but you should eat until full. The fasting period ensures that you burn through quite a bit of your stored energy, and deliberately trying to cut calories further is often difficult in the long term.

The 5:2 Diet

A related approach is the 5:2 diet championed by Dr. Michael Mosley, a TV producer and physician based in the UK, where his book *The Fast Diet* was a best-seller. Rather than completely abstaining from food for a period of time, this diet calls for a period of low caloric intake. However, the calories are kept low enough to trigger many of the same beneficial hormonal adaptations as fasting. There are many anecdotes of success with this method.

The 5:2 diet consists of five normal eating days. On the other two "fast" days, women may eat up to 500 calories per day and men up to 600 calories. These two fast days can be done on consecutive days or spaced apart, depending upon your preference. The 500 to 600 calories can be consumed in a single meal or spread out into multiple meals over the course of a day (though of course they would be very small meals).

The reason a limited number of calories are allowed on fast days is to increase compliance. Dr. Mosley felt that taking no calories at all during a day was excessively difficult, to the point that many people simply couldn't do it. While I've found that people are more capable of fasting than they may think, the 5:2 diet can be a good way to ease into fasting. The 5:2 diet is generally followed indefinitely, even after target weight is reached, in order to maintain weight loss.

> Three 24-hour fasts spread throughout the week works for me. It's actually not a big deal merely missing a meal or two. And I know that most of the fast happens when I am sleeping. I eat my meal in the evening on the fast day and it's interesting to note that I enjoy it so much more because I am properly hungry—just as nature intended.
>
> **—Stella B., Leeds, UK**

MARK SISSON ▮ FASTING ALL-STARS

If someone had a serious amount of weight to lose and had spent the requisite time teaching their body to burn fat, I would have them try 24-, 36-, and 48-hour fasts. Probably not much longer than that, but probably with some frequency (2 days every week or every 2 weeks, for 6 weeks, and then rest). As long as they were exercising and performing substantial movement throughout the day, they would be burning fat, utilizing ketones, and possibly even building muscle.

Alternate-Day Fasting

As the name suggests, in alternate-day fasting, you fast every other day. As on the 5:2 diet, 500 to 600 calories are permitted on each fasting day, but because fasting is done every other day rather than twice per week, it's a slightly more intense regimen than the 5:2 diet. This regimen should be followed until you reach target weight. After that, the number of fasting days can be reduced as long as you're maintaining the ideal weight.

Leonie Heilbronn, in searching for an alternative to daily caloric restriction, tested the feasibility of using alternate-day fasting for weight loss. Testing this regimen on men and women volunteers proved that weight loss could be sustained.

Krista Varady, an assistant professor of nutrition at the University of Chicago, confirmed the efficacy and validity of this fasting schedule in a study she performed in 2010. She guided men and women through an alternate-day fasting protocol for one month. After that, they continued with the protocol on their own for the next thirty days. At the end of those thirty days (two months total on the protocol), weight loss averaged 12.6 pounds. Importantly, lean mass (muscle, protein, and bone) remained unchanged—that weight loss was purely due to loss of fat.

Just do what you can depending on your mindset and stress levels at the time, and never be disappointed if you "snap." Think of it as turning off the "food switch" in your mind for as long as you can.

—**Dianne D.,
Norfolk, UK**

FASTING ALL-STARS ROBB WOLF

Longer fasting seems best approached when you have some downtime and can control your activity, work demands, etc. From the ancestral perspective, fasting is almost certainly a key piece of our genetic heritage. That said, we tend to have more chronic stress and demands than what would typify the ancestral environment. So I think it's important to keep an eye on allostatic load when considering what duration of fast one might tackle.

36-Hour Fasts

In a thirty-six-hour fast, you do not eat for one entire day. For example, if you finish dinner at 7 p.m. on day 1, your fast would begin immediately after— you skip all meals on day 2 and not eat again until breakfast at 7 a.m. on day 3. That totals thirty-six hours of fasting.

In our IDM Program, we use thirty-six-hour fasts, on a three-times-a-week schedule, with patients who have type 2 diabetes. We continue this schedule until the desired results are achieved: the patient is able to go off of all diabetes medication and has reached the desired weight. After that, we reduce the frequency of fasting to a level that lets the patient maintain the hard-won gains but is easier on the patient. How long the three-times-a-week schedule is maintained varies, but in general, the longer the patient has had diabetes, the longer the duration of fasting required. We cannot reverse twenty years of diabetes in a few weeks. But the longer-duration fasting period gives us the needed power to get good results in a reasonable time.

DR. MICHAEL RUSCIO █FASTING ALL-STARS

Most of my patients feel best when they start with a longer fast of 2–4 days to get their gastrointestinal symptoms under control. Then they can periodically fast for a half day or full day as needed for maintenance, maybe once a week or a few times a week. The more severe someone's symptoms are, the more likely I am to recommend a longer fast, but the longer fasts contain some type of liquid nutrition, such as broth or semi-elemental nutrition. The main concerns are fatigue, weight loss, and nutrient depletion, but these can be safeguarded against by using a good liquid formula like a semi-elemental diet.

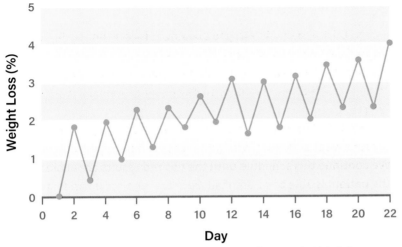

Figure 13.1. Alternate-day fasting results in steady weight loss. The valleys represent fed days, when weight goes back up slightly.

Source: Heilbronn et al., "Alternate-Day Fasting in Nonobese Subjects: Effects on Body Weight, Body Composition, and Energy Metabolism."

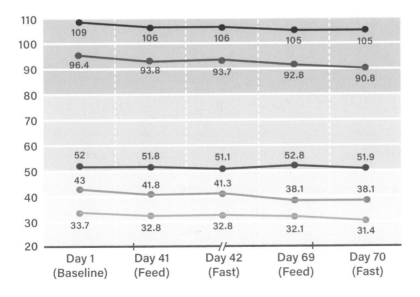

Figure 13.2. Over two months of alternate-day fasting, body weight, BMI, body fat, and waist circumference all declined, but there was no loss of fat-free mass (muscle and bone).

- ● Body weight (kg)
- ● BMI (kg/m²)
- ● Fat mass (kg)
- ● Fat-free mass (kg)
- ● Waist circumference (cm)

Source: Bhutani et al., "Improvements in Coronary Heart Disease Risk Indicators by Alternate-Day Fasting Involve Adipose Tissue Modulations."

We recommend that blood sugar be checked regularly between two and four times per day, as there is the potential for low blood sugar as well as high blood sugar. Medications are generally reduced on the fasting day to prevent hypoglycemia—again, talk to your doctor if you're on medication before trying a fasting regimen. However, since changes in medication affect everyone slightly differently, there is the possibility of reducing medications too much, resulting in high blood sugar. Testing regularly allows you to fine-tune the medication so you're getting just as much as you need, no more, no less.

42-Hour Fasts

Many clients in the IDM Program routinely skip the morning meal and have their first meal of the day around noon. This makes it easy to follow a sixteen-hour fasting regimen (see page 203) on regular days. There is nothing magical about eating as soon as you get up. Starting the day with just a large cup of coffee is quite acceptable.

Combining this daily routine with an occasional (two to three times per week) thirty-six-hour fast results in a forty-two-hour fasting period. For example, you would eat dinner at 6 p.m. on day 1. You skip all meals on day 2 and eat your regular "breakfast" meal at noon on day 3. This gives you a total fast of forty-two hours.

References

Alison Fildes, Judith Charlton, Caroline Rudisill, Peter Littlejohns, A. Toby Prevost, and Martin C. Gulliford, "Probability of an Obese Person Attaining Normal Body Weight: Cohort Study Using Electronic Health Records," *American Journal of Public Health* 105, no. 9 (2015): e54–e59.

Leonie K. Heilbronn, Steven R. Smith, Corby K. Martin, Stephen D. Anton, and Eric Ravussin, "Alternate-Day Fasting in Nonobese Subjects: Effects on Body Weight, Body Composition, and Energy Metabolism," *American Journal of Clinical Nutrition* 81, no. 1 (2005): 69–73.

Surabhi Bhutani, Monica C. Klempel, Reed A. Berger, and Krista A. Varady, "Improvements in Coronary Heart Disease Risk Indicators by Alternate-Day Fasting Involve Adipose Tissue Modulations," *Obesity* 18, no. 11 (2010): 2152–9.

SUNNY & CHERRIE

FASTING SUCCESS STORY

I first met Sunny in September 2015 in the Intensive Dietary Management Program. Sunny, age fifty-one, had been diagnosed with type 2 diabetes in the mid-1990s, when he was only in his thirties, and had been started on the medication metformin. Over the years, he'd required more and more medications to control his blood sugar levels. In 2011 he was prescribed insulin. By the time I saw him, he was taking maximal doses of metformin in addition to injecting 70 units of insulin every day.

Despite this large dose of medication, his blood sugar was still suboptimally controlled; his HbA1C, which reflects the three-month average blood sugar level, was 7.2 percent. Optimal blood sugar control is defined as less than 7.0 percent, although many physicians recommend getting it to less than 6.5 percent.

Sunny started participating in our IDM Program on October 2, 2015. He changed to a diet low in refined carbohydrates and high in natural fats. In addition, we asked him to fast for thirty-six to forty-two hours three times a week. If he finished dinner on day 1, he would not eat again until lunch on day 3.

His blood sugar improved immediately. In just two weeks, we were able to discontinue all of his insulin. One month after that, we stopped all his diabetic medications entirely. He has since maintained normal blood sugar without any medications, managed entirely by dietary measures.

Over the Christmas holiday period, he, like many patients in our program, did gain weight and his blood sugar did increase slightly. However, with the resumption of his diet and intermittent fasting, his weight and blood sugar fell back down, and he did not require medications.

Sunny felt remarkably well throughout his entire journey. He had no difficulty maintaining his low-carbohydrate diet or the intermittent fasting protocols. By March 2016, his weight had stabilized and his body mass index was only 19.

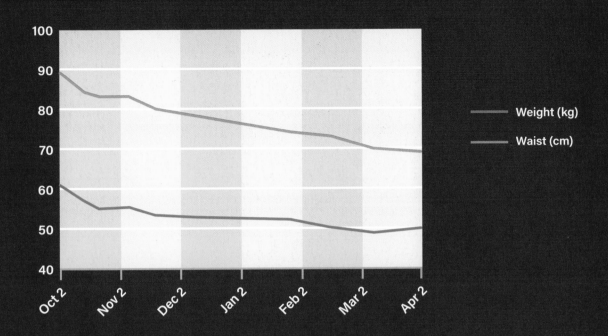

Weight (kg)	Waist (cm)

More importantly, his waist size had come down dramatically. Waist size is a good reflection of how much visceral fat around the organs of the abdomen and therefore more accurately reflects the body's metabolic state. The waist/hip ratio and waist/height ratio are considered better predictors of health than simple body weight.

Even more remarkably, Sunny's kidney function improved right away on the program. When he started the fasting regimen, he was spilling protein in his urine, well above the normal limit. This protein in the urine is the first sign of diabetic damage to the kidney and is often considered irreversible, just as type 2 diabetes itself is considered irreversible. But by November, just a month after he started fasting, his protein excretion had fallen to well within the normal range, where it has remained ever since.

In March 2016, Sunny did not need to lose any more weight, so his fasting regimen was reduced to twenty-four hours of fasting three times a week for maintenance. Of course, if he had dietary indiscretions or if his blood sugar or weight started to rise, he could easily increase his fasting days as needed.

After injecting himself with insulin twice daily for five years and taking diabetic medications for over twenty years, Sunny was free of type 2 diabetes, with just a few short months of proper diet and intermittent fasting. His blood sugar levels now classify him as prediabetic, not a full-fledged diabetic. His disease had reversed.

But that is not the end of the story.

Cherrie

In January 2016, Sunny's older sister Cherrie was astonished at how well her younger brother was doing. His weight was down. His waist size was down. He had stopped all his diabetic medications. He didn't even find the lifestyle change very difficult. His twenty years of diabetes had been reversed almost overnight. Cherrie wanted in.

Cherrie was fifty-five years old and had been diagnosed with type 2 diabetes nine years earlier at age forty-six. Her story was similar to her brother's: she had started off with a small dose of a single medication for diabetes, but over the years, her medication pile had slowly grown. She was now taking three medications for diabetes, along with medication for cholesterol, blood pressure, and heartburn.

We discussed her situation and together decided upon a dietary plan for her. She would change to a diet low in refined carbohydrates and high in natural fats. She was a little less sure of how she would feel during fasting, so we decided upon a twenty-four-hour fasting period three times per week. Her diabetes was not as severe as her brother's, and she could always increase her fasting if necessary.

She started our program in February 2016. Her blood sugar levels responded immediately. Within two weeks, she had stopped all three of her diabetic medications, as they were no longer necessary. Her blood sugar was now consistently in the normal range. Her weight began a steady decline, as did her waist size.

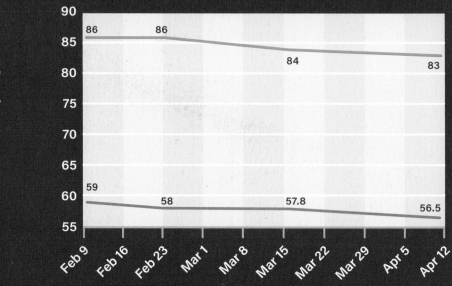

Her heartburn disappeared, so she stopped her heartburn medication. Her blood pressure normalized, so she stopped her blood pressure medication. Her cholesterol numbers were improved, so she stopped her cholesterol medications. Within a single month, she stopped all six of her medications, yet her bloodwork was better than ever. Her HbA1c of 6.2 percent was better than when she was taking all three diabetes medications. She was no longer considered diabetic, only prediabetic. This meant that her disease was reversing.

Furthermore, she felt extremely well during this entire process. She did not have any trouble with the fasting protocol. While her fasting period was shorter than Sunny's, she was still getting excellent results, so there was no need to change it. She had been taking six medications at the beginning. Now she was on none, and she felt a hundred times better.

This illustrates an important point. Type 2 diabetes is a dietary disease. As such, the only logical treatment is to change diet and lifestyle.

If the problem stems from an excessive intake of carbohydrates, then reducing carbohydrates is the answer. If the problem stems from excessive weight, then successful weight loss with fasting is the answer. Once we fix the underlying issue, the disease reverses.

However, we have been brainwashed to believe that type 2 diabetes and all its complications are inevitable. We have been deceived into believing that we can successfully treat a dietary disease with increasing doses of drugs. When the drugs fail to halt the diabetes, we are told that the disease is chronic and progressive.

Sunny had type 2 diabetes for over twenty years, yet he managed to successfully reverse his disease within a matter of months. Cherrie had been on diabetes medication for seven years and also successfully reversed her disease in a few months. But they are not anomalies. Almost every single day, I meet people of all ages who have reversed or are reversing their type 2 diabetes with a fasting regimen.

Chapter 14
EXTENDED FASTING

Extended fasts—those lasting longer than forty-two hours—have been followed for centuries in cultures all over the world. They have also been extensively studied in the medical literature as far back as 1915, when doctors Otto Folin and W. Denis described fasting as a "safe and effective method for reducing the weight of those suffering from obesity"; they were echoed by Francis Gano Benedict in the same year in his book on prolonged fasting. But thereafter, interest in extended fasting as a therapeutic tool seemed to fade away.

Interest revived in the late 1950s and 1960s as more and more physicians reported their experiences with fasting. Early studies focused mostly on shorter fasting periods, but once they became more familiar with fasting, many physicians extended the fasts.

In 1968, endocrinologist Ian Gilliland studied the effects of extended fasting on forty-six patients. After admitting them to the hospital for observation to make sure they were compliant with the fast, he initiated a fourteen-day fast during which they were allowed only water, tea, and coffee. After that, they were discharged and asked to follow a 600- to 1000-calorie diet at home. Interestingly, two patients asked to be readmitted for a second fourteen-day period of fasting. Having gotten good results already with relative ease, they wanted even better results by increasing the duration of the fast.

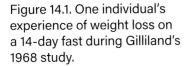

Figure 14.1. One individual's experience of weight loss on a 14-day fast during Gilliland's 1968 study.

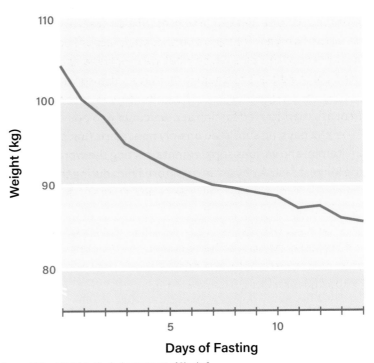

Source: Gilliland, "Total Fasting in the Treatment of Obesity."

After fourteen days of fasting, the average weight loss was 17.2 pounds. Blood sugar levels fell during fasting, as expected, to levels that significantly benefited the participants with diabetes—all three diabetic patients were completely off insulin by the end of the two weeks.

Insulin encourages the kidneys to retain salt and water, so by lowering insulin levels, fasting helps the body excrete excess salt and water. During the first several days of fasting, there's a corresponding increase in urine flow. The elimination of excess water and salt helped one patient in Gilliland's study who had severe congestive heart failure: by the end of the two weeks, he was able to walk without breathlessness.

Was fasting for two weeks hard? Quite the opposite, in fact. Gilliland describes the participants having a "feeling of well being" and "euphoria." Were they hungry? Perhaps surprisingly, not really: "We did not encounter complaints of hunger after the first day." These experiences were confirmed by other researchers of the time.

However, the study participants didn't do so well following the 600- to 1000-calorie diet Gilliland prescribed once they were sent home. In the two-year follow-up period, 50 percent of participants did not adhere to this diet. Given what we now know about reduced-calorie diets (see Chapter 5), that's not surprising.

Fasting has no upper limit. In the 1970s, a twenty-seven-year-old Scottish man started fasting at a weight of 456 pounds. Over the next 382 days, he subsisted on only noncaloric fluids, a daily multivitamin, and various supplements, setting the world record for the longest fast. A physician monitored him during the fasting period and determined that there were no significant deleterious health effects.

His body weight decreased from 456 pounds to 180 pounds. Even five years after his fast, he remained at 196 pounds. His blood sugar level decreased but remained well within the normal range, and he had no episodes of hypoglycemia.

What to Expect During an Extended Fast

In Gilliland's study, forty-four of forty-six patients completed the two-week fasting period. One developed nausea and one simply decided against it and dropped out. That's a 96 percent completion rate! Even a two-week fast is not as difficult as many think. Our clinical experience confirms this: people often believe they cannot fast, but once we explain the process, give helpful tips for success, and provide proper support, patients in the IDM Program quickly realize that fasting is actually quite easy.

That's not to say that there's not an adjustment period. In fact, the first several days of fasting are often quite difficult. Day 2 seems to be the hardest in terms of hunger. However, once you push through that second day, things get progressively easier. Hunger slowly disappears and a sense of well-being often develops. It's just like exercising. When you first start to lift weights, for example, your muscles are very sore afterward. This is expected and should not dissuade you from continuing to work out—and over time, as you grow stronger, you can lift the same weight without difficulty or soreness. Similarly, with fasting, the initial period may also be difficult, but things get easier with practice.

I fast 3.5 consecutive days a week and eat LCHF the other 3.5 days. It has been working very well! It is my version of an alternate-day pattern but in blocks instead. I love that Dr. Fung encourages experimentation to find a pattern that works for each unique individual.

—Evelyn C., Regina, SK

Weight loss averaged 0.76 pounds per day in Dr. Gilliland's study, adjusting for the expected water-weight regain once the fast was completed. Other studies of fasting for over two hundred days show similar rates of weight loss, ranging from 0.41 to 0.67 pounds per day. In the IDM Program, we tell patients to expect an average fat loss of half a pound per day of fasting. If you lose more weight than that, it's likely water weight that you're shedding due to the reduction in insulin.

If we assume that 2,000 calories are burned during a normal day, and we know that one pound of fat contains approximately 3,500 calories, then during an absolute fast—when no calories at all are being consumed—we would expect 0.57 pounds to be lost each day (2,000 calories expended / 3,500 calories per pound = 0.57 pounds lost). That's fairly close to what studies have shown. This means that metabolism stays relatively stable throughout the fasting period—there's no metabolic slowdown, so those 2,000 calories that are burned on a normal day are also burned during fasting. So, for a patient with 100 pounds of fat, you can expect that it would take roughly 200 full days of fasting to lose it all.

During extended fasting, the brain reduces its reliance on glucose as an energy source. Instead, the majority of the brain's fuel is supplied by ketone bodies, which are created by burning fat. It is believed that the brain is able to more efficiently use these ketones, possibly leading to improved mental abilities. Ketones have sometimes been referred to as a "superfuel" for the brain. Ketones generally require thirty-six to forty-eight hours of fasting to ramp up. Prior to this, most of the body's energy requirements are met by the breakdown of glycogen. (See page 44 for more details.)

Extended fasting rarely causes electrolyte abnormalities. Calcium, phosphorus, sodium, potassium, chloride urea, creatinine, and bicarbonate levels in the blood remain within the normal limits and are virtually unchanged by the end of the fast. Blood magnesium levels occasionally go low. This seems to be especially prevalent in diabetics. Most of the body's magnesium is intracellular and not measured by blood levels. While monitoring the world-record-breaking 382-day fast, researchers measured the

Incorporating intermittent fasting (16:8 and 20:4) and heavy lifting / interval training (to preserve muscle mass and drain those glucose stores) helped me get into ketosis faster and lose fat more efficiently than using a well-formulated ketogenic diet alone. Diet alone takes about 3+ weeks to get past hunger, but fasting and exercise with keto cuts time in half.

—Leslie E.,
Venice, FL

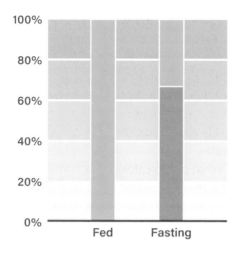

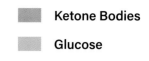

Figure 14.2. After a fast of several weeks, the brain is fueled primarily by ketones.

Source: Cahill, "Fuel Metabolism in Starvation."

magnesium content within the cells, which remained firmly in the normal range. Nevertheless, we often supplement patients with magnesium to be on the safe side.

It's normal for bowel movements to slow down during prolonged fasting—nothing goes into the digestive system, so it makes sense that little comes out. During the world-record fast, bowel movements occurred every thirty-seven to forty-eight days. It's important to note that this is an entirely normal phenomenon. You do not *need* to have a daily bowel movement to feel well. Discomfort from constipation occurs when your intestines are full of stool, but during an extended fast, there is little inside the colon and therefore little discomfort. This also reflects the fact that the body is recycling all the essential fats and amino acids from the breakdown of old or dysfunctional cells.

Finally, one more cautionary note for those who have diabetes and/or are taking medications: you *must* talk to your physician before starting any prolonged fasting. Also, if you feel unwell at any point during the fasting, you must stop. You may feel hungry, but you should not feel faint, unwell, or nauseated. This is not normal, and you should not attempt to push through.

Two- to Three-Day Fasts

When dealing with stubborn weight plateaus or persistently high blood sugar, one option is to simply extend the fasting period for longer than forty-two hours. How long to continue the fast is a matter of personal preference. However, there are some general guidelines we can offer.

In the IDM Program, we rarely advise patients to use fasting durations of two to three days. The majority of people find day 2 of an extended fast to be the most difficult in terms of hunger. After day 2, many people describe a gradual lessening and then a total elimination of hunger. (Some have hypothesized that this effect is due to the high number of ketone bodies that begin circulating after a couple of days.) From a practical standpoint, it seems rather harsh to end a fast as soon as you have passed its most difficult day. Instead, we encourage patients to continue their fast for seven to fourteen days. A fourteen-day fast delivers seven times the benefit of a two-day fast but is only marginally more difficult.

Seven- to Fourteen-Day Fasts

We often start patients with severe type 2 diabetes on a seven- to fourteen-day fast. There are several reasons for this. First, it allows the body to quickly adjust to fasting conditions, which many people find easier than a more gradual transition. It is really the difference between doing a cannonball jump into the deep end of the pool and gradually wading in, one inch at a time. For some, the cannonball is the easier choice.

Second, the longer fasting period allows for more rapid improvements in blood glucose and type 2 diabetes. In patients on high doses of medication or who are suffering the complications of organ damage, there is a more urgent need to reverse the diabetes and lose weight—much of the organ damage caused by diabetes is irreversible once it occurs. It's often not until day 5 or 6 that we see significant improvement in blood sugar and are able to reduce the diabetes medication. This result would take much longer using a shorter fasting duration.

We generally cap the duration of a fast at fourteen days in order to minimize the risk of refeeding syndrome (see below). However, many people have extended their fasts well past fourteen days without incident. In general, though, we advise patients to switch to an alternate-day fasting regimen for two weeks before repeating an extended fast.

Refeeding Syndrome

Refeeding refers to the one to two days immediately after an extended fast. Medical complications during refeeding were first described in severely malnourished Americans in Japanese prisoner of war camps after World War II. Since then, refeeding syndrome has also been described upon treatment of longstanding anorexia nervosa and of alcoholic patients. It is particularly prone to occur in these groups of patients because they are often malnourished and do not have significant body fat stores to begin with. During the ensuing long periods without food, their bodies may break down functional proteins to supply much-needed energy. This syndrome is extremely uncommon in patients with adequate body fat stores who are well-nourished. But even then, it may occur rarely if you are attempting an extended fast—typically greater than five days at a time.

Refeeding syndrome occurs when electrolytes, particularly phosphorus, are depleted due to malnourishment. Adults store 500 to 800 grams of phosphorus in the body. Approximately 80 percent of that is held within the skeleton, the rest in soft tissues. Most phosphorus is kept inside the tissue cells rather than in the blood, and the blood level of phosphorus is very tightly controlled. During prolonged malnutrition, blood levels of phosphorus remain normal as bone stores are used up.

Once refeeding begins, the food raises insulin levels, which stimulates the synthesis of glycogen, fat, and protein. All of that requires minerals like phosphorus and magnesium. This puts an enormous demand on already-depleted phosphorus stores. Too little phosphorus is left in the blood, and that causes the body to "power down." Muscle weakness and outright muscle breakdown have been described. It may even affect the heart muscle and the diaphragm, the muscle responsible for breathing.

Magnesium can also become depleted, resulting in cramps, confusion, tremor, and, occasionally, seizures. Low potassium and magnesium can also cause heart rhythm disturbances or even outright cardiac arrest. In addition, higher insulin levels during refeeding may occasionally cause the kidneys to retain salt and water. This may show up as swelling of the feet and ankles and has been termed refeeding edema.

Chronically malnourished and/or severely underweight people are at the highest risk of refeeding syndrome. This includes those with anorexia, chronic alcoholism, cancer, uncontrolled diabetes, or bowel disease—if any of these apply to you, fasting may not be for you; discuss your options with your doctor. And more generally, people with a body mass index less than 18.5, unintentional weight loss of more than 10 percent of their body weight in the past six months, or a history of alcoholism or misuse of drugs should be especially careful about extended fasting. These groups of patients are generally malnourished and underweight rather than overweight, so there's no reason to try fasting as a therapeutic tool. However, if absolutely necessary (for example, religious or spiritual purposes), they may consider shorter-term fasts lasting less than twenty-four hours.

Fortunately, refeeding syndrome is very rare. Even among very sick hospitalized patients, studies found it occurred in only 0.43 percent. The main risk factor for refeeding syndrome is prolonged malnutrition. When we use fasting as a therapeutic tool in our IDM clinic, most people have never missed a single meal in over twenty-five years! Malnutrition is definitely not a concern.

Refeeding syndrome occurs mostly when people have been starved—that is, they've undergone an uncontrolled, involuntary restriction of food—and particularly when they've begun wasting (experiencing severe malnutrition due to starvation). Refeeding syndrome due to fasting—that is, the controlled, voluntary restriction of food—is very uncommon.

To help prevent problems in the post-fast refeeding period, there are two steps we recommend:

1. Do not make an extended fast a water-only fast. Drinking homemade bone broth provides phosphorus and other proteins and electrolytes, which reduces the chances of developing refeeding syndrome. And to prevent vitamin deficiency, take a daily multivitamin.

2. Do all your usual activities, especially your exercise program, during your fast. This helps to maintain your muscles and bones.

In 2003, the performance artist David Blaine underwent a forty-four-day water-only fast. He lost 54 pounds (24.5 kg), a massive 25 percent of his body weight. His body mass index dropped from 29 to 21.6. While his blood sugar and cholesterol levels remained normal, he developed refeeding syndrome and edema.

David Blaine was suspended in a Plexiglas box for the duration of his fast. He could not do any of his usual activities, or even stand up, for forty-four days. This is far more than a fast. His muscles and bones actually developed significant atrophy during that period. He was losing far more than fat: he lost significant lean weight, muscle and bone. This was not due to fasting but instead to being cooped up in a box for forty-four days.

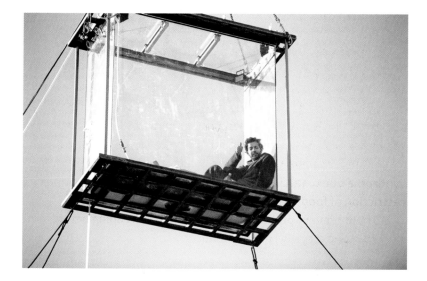

In 2003, David Blaine underwent a 44-day water-only fast suspended in a Plexiglas box above London.

References

Ernst J. Drenick, Marion E. Swendseid, William H. Blahd, and Stewart G. Tuttle, "Prolonged Starvation as Treatment for Severe Obesity," *JAMA* 187, no. 2 (1964): 100–5.

Francis Gano Benedict, *A Study of Prolonged Fasting* (Washington, DC: Carnegie Institute of Washington, 1915): 27, 42, 182.

George F. Cahill Jr., "Fuel Metabolism in Starvation," *Annual Review of Nutrition* 26 (2006): 1–22.

I. C. Gilliland, "Total Fasting in the Treatment of Obesity," *Postgraduate Medical Journal* 44, no. 507 (1968): 58–61.

M. A. Camp and M. Allon, "Severe Hypophosphatemia in Hospitalized Patients," *Mineral and Electrolyte Metabolism* 16, no. 6 (1990): 365-8.

M. A. Crook, V. Hally, and J. V. Panteli, "The Importance of the Refeeding Syndrome," *Nutrition* 17, nos. 7–8 (2001): 632–7.

Otto Folin and W. Denis, "On Starvation and Obesity, with Special Reference to Acidosis," *Journal of Biological Chemistry* 21 (1915): 183–92.

W. K. Steward and Laura W. Fleming, "Features of a Successful Therapeutic Fast of 382 Days' Duration," *Postgraduate Medical Journal* 49, no. 569 (1973): 203–9.

Chapter 15
FASTING TIPS AND FAQS

Fasting used to be an integral part of normal life. In fact, it still is in many religions—for example, the Greek Orthodox and Muslim religions. In these contexts, it's a communal practice. You're not fasting alone but with all of your family and friends. Peer support is widely available, and practical tips are passed on from generation to generation. However, with the decline in the practice of fasting, good advice is often difficult to find.

In this chapter, we'll present practical tips and answer common questions based on our experiences with hundreds of fasting patients.

But first, two general suggestions for fasting success: One, always keep your goals in mind. For example, if you are trying to lose several pounds for an upcoming class reunion, your fasting strategy will be different than if you are 400 pounds and severely diabetic.

Two, readjust your strategy based on your results. If you follow a regimen of alternate-day fasting and get good results, great! But if your progress stalls, then it may be a good idea to change paths. If you find longer fasts much easier than shorter ones, then adjust your regimen to add longer fasts into your fasting schedule. Or you may find shorter, more-frequent fasts better in the summer and longer, less-frequent fasts better in the winter. Adjust and adapt. Nothing is written in stone.

Top 9 Fasting Tips

1. Drink water: Start each morning with a full eight-ounce glass of water. It will help you start your day hydrated and set the tone for drinking plenty of fluids throughout the day.

2. Stay busy: It'll keep your mind off food. Try fasting on a busy workday. You may be too busy to remember to be hungry.

3. Drink coffee: Coffee is a mild appetite suppressant. There's also some evidence that green tea may suppress appetite. Black tea and homemade bone broth may also help control appetite.

4. Ride the waves: Hunger comes in waves; it is not constant. When it hits, slowly drink a glass of water or a hot cup of coffee. Often by the time you've finished, your hunger will have passed.

5. Don't tell people you are fasting: Most people will try to discourage you simply because they don't understand the benefits of fasting. A close-knit support group of people who are also fasting is often beneficial, but telling everybody you know is not a good idea.

6. Give yourself one month: It takes time for your body to get used to fasting. The first few times you fast will be difficult, so be prepared. Don't be discouraged. It gets easier.

7. Follow a nutritious diet on nonfasting days: Intermittent fasting is not an excuse to eat whatever you like. During nonfasting days, stick to a nutritious diet low in sugar and refined carbohydrates. Following a low-carbohydrate diet that's high in healthy fats can also help your body stay in fat-burning mode and make fasting easier.

8. Don't binge: After your fast, pretend it never happened. Eat normally (and nutritiously—see #7), as if you had never fasted.

9. Fit fasting into your own life: This is the most important tip I can offer, and it has the greatest impact on whether you stick to your fasting regimen. Do not change your life to fit your fasting schedule—change your fasting schedule to fit your life. Don't limit yourself socially because you're fasting. There will be times during which it's impossible to fast, such as vacations, holidays, and weddings. Do not try to force fasting into these celebrations. These occasions are times to relax and enjoy. Afterwards, you can simply increase your fasting to compensate. Or just resume your regular fasting schedule. Adjust your fasting schedule to what makes sense for your lifestyle. We'll talk more about this on page 246.

Fasting is no different than any other skill in life: practice and support are essential to performing it well.

Breaking Your Fast

Break your fast gently. The longer the fasting period, the gentler you must be. There is a natural tendency to overeat as soon as the fast is over—though, interestingly, most people say that this isn't because of overwhelming hunger but more of a psychological need to eat. Overeating right after fasting often leads to stomach discomfort. While not serious, it can be quite uncomfortable. This problem tends to be self-correcting.

Try breaking your fast with a snack or small dish to start, then wait for thirty to sixty minutes before eating your main meal. This will usually give time for any waves of hunger to pass and allow you to gradually adjust to eating again. Short-duration fasts (twenty-four hours or less) generally require no special precautions, but for longer fasts, it is a good idea to plan ahead. Prepare a small dish and leave it in the refrigerator so that when it comes time to break the fast, you are ready and less likely to be tempted by the myriad of other convenience foods available. Here are some suggestions for that first snack:

> ¼ to ⅓ cup macadamia nuts, almonds, walnuts, or pine nuts
>
> 1 tablespoon peanut butter or almond butter
>
> A small salad (instead of salad dressing, try cottage cheese or crème fraîche)
>
> A small bowl of raw vegetables with some olive oil and vinegar drizzled on them
>
> A bowl of vegetable soup
>
> A small amount of meat (for instance, three slices of prosciutto or a slice or two of pork belly)

For those who experience gastrointestinal distress when breaking a fast, eggs seem to be the biggest culprit. If you have a sensitive stomach or are concerned about breaking your fast, you may want to avoid eggs at your first meal.

Tips for Breaking Your Fast with a Snack

- Make sure your portion sizes are small. You will be eating a full meal shortly, so there is no need to gorge.
- Take the time to chew thoroughly. This will greatly help your digestive system, which has been resting for a while. You are slowly bringing your system back online.
- Take your time in general. Your fast is over. If you are feeling anxious to eat again, take comfort knowing you will be having a whole meal within the hour.
- Don't forget to drink water! Drink a tall glass of water before you break your fast and after your first meal. People often forget to consume fluid once they stop fasting, but we often mistake thirst for hunger. Make sure you are staying hydrated so you don't overeat.

Common Concerns

Hunger

This is probably the number-one concern people have about fasting. They assume they'll be overwhelmed with hunger and unable to control themselves during the fast. We've devoted Chapter 9 to hunger, debunking myths and explaining how it really works, but here, we offer a quick overview of what you can expect in terms of hunger and what can help minimize it.

The truth is that hunger does not persist but instead comes in waves. If you're experiencing hunger, it will pass. Staying busy during a fast day is often helpful.

As the body becomes accustomed to fasting, it starts to burn its stores of fat, which helps suppress hunger. Many people note that over several weeks, as they continue a fasting regimen, appetite not only doesn't increase, it actually starts to *decrease*. During longer fasts, many people notice that their hunger completely disappears by the second or third day.

There are some drinks or spices allowed on fasts that can help suppress hunger. Here are my top five natural appetite suppressants:

Water: Start your day with a full glass of cold water. Staying hydrated helps prevent hunger. (Drinking a glass of water prior to a meal may also reduce hunger and help prevent overeating.) Sparkling mineral water may help for noisy stomachs and cramping.

Green tea: Full of antioxidants and polyphenols, green tea is a great aid for dieters. The powerful antioxidants may help stimulate metabolism and weight loss.

Cinnamon: Cinnamon has been shown to slow gastric emptying and may help suppress hunger. It may also help lower blood sugar and therefore is useful in weight loss. Cinnamon may be added to all teas and coffees for a delicious change of pace.

Coffee: While many assume that it is the caffeine in coffee that suppresses hunger, studies show that this effect is more likely related to antioxidants—although caffeine may raise your metabolism, further boosting fat-burning. But a study shows that both decaffeinated and regular coffee suppress hunger better than caffeine in water. Given its health benefits, there is no reason to limit coffee intake.

Chia seeds: Chia seeds are high in soluble fiber and omega-3 fatty acids. These seeds absorb water and form a gel when soaked in liquid for thirty minutes, which may aid in appetite suppression. They can be eaten dry or made into a gel or pudding. These may be taken during a fast to help suppress hunger. Once again, while technically breaking the fast, the effect is so slight that it does not significantly detract from the benefits of the fast. The increased compliance more than compensates.

For more on hunger, see Chapter 9.

Dizziness

If you experience dizziness during your fast, most likely, you're becoming dehydrated. Preventing this requires both salt and water. Be sure to drink plenty of fluids, and in case you're low on salt, add extra sea salt to homemade bone broth or mineral water.

Another possibility is that your blood pressure is too low—particularly if you're taking medications for hypertension. Speak to your physician about adjusting your medication.

Headaches

Headaches are common the first few times you fast. It is believed that they're caused by the transition from a relatively high-salt diet to very low salt intake on fasting days. Headaches are usually temporary, and as you become accustomed to fasting, this problem often resolves itself. In the meantime, take some extra salt in the form of broth or mineral water.

Constipation

This is common and to be expected. Bowel movements will typically decrease during a fast simply because there is less food intake. If you are not experiencing actual discomfort, then there's no need to worry about decreased bowel movements.

However, increasing your intake of fiber, fruits, and vegetables during the nonfasting period may help with constipation.

I was unable to water fast in the past due to severe nausea and weakness. Now I've successfully completed a 7-day water-only fast for 7 days by adding 1 teaspoon of salt to a glass of water daily. I felt wonderful, with no nausea or weakness!

—Cinda H., Colorado

Metamucil can also be taken during or after fasting to increase fiber and stool bulk. If the problem continues, ask your doctor to consider prescribing a laxative.

Heartburn

To prevent heartburn after a fast, avoid taking large meals—try to just eat normally. Avoiding lying down immediately after a meal can also help; try to stay in an upright position for at least a half hour after meals. Similarly, placing wooden blocks under the head of your bed to raise it may help with nighttime symptoms. In addition, drinking sparkling water with lemon often helps. If none of these options work for you, consult your physician.

Muscle Cramps

Low magnesium, which is particularly common in diabetics, may cause muscle cramps. You may take an over-the-counter magnesium supplement. You may also soak in Epsom salts, which are magnesium salts. Add a cup to a warm bath and soak in it for half an hour—the magnesium will be absorbed through your skin. Alternatively, you may look for magnesium oil, which also allows magnesium to be absorbed through the skin.

FAQs

Will fasting make me cranky?

Interestingly, this has not been a problem in our Intensive Dietary Management Program, despite years of experience and hundreds of patients. Similarly, members of religions that embrace routine fasting are not known to be cranky. For example, nobody would stereotype a Buddhist monk, who engages in fasting almost daily, as a cranky guy. I think that when people become irritable when they don't eat, it's because they *expect* to be cranky, so they act out their role in a self-fulfilling prophecy. When we normalize the idea of fasting in their minds, they forget to become cranky.

Will fasting make me tired?

No. In our experience at the Intensive Dietary Management Program, the opposite is true. Many people find that they have more energy during a fast—probably due to increased adrenaline. You'll find that you have plenty of energy for all the normal activities of daily living. Persistent fatigue is not a normal part of fasting. If you experience excessive fatigue, you should stop fasting immediately and see your doctor.

Will fasting make me confused or forgetful?

No. You should not experience any decrease in memory or concentration during your fast. On the contrary, fasting improves mental clarity and acuity. Over the long term, fasting may actually help improve memory. One theory is that fasting activates a form of cellular cleansing called autophagy that may help prevent age-associated memory loss—see page 151 for more.

Does fasting lead to overeating?

The simple answer is yes, you will eat more than usual immediately after fasting. However, the amount of food eaten above the baseline on nonfasting days is not enough to offset the preceding fast. A study of thirty-six-hour fasts shows that the meal taken after the fast is almost 20 percent larger than usual, but over the entire two-day period, there was still a net deficit of 1,958 calories. The amount "overeaten" did not nearly compensate for the fast. The study concludes, "A 36-hour fast . . . did not induce a powerful, unconditioned stimulus to compensate on the subsequent day."

My stomach is always growling. What can I do?

Try drinking some mineral water. The mechanism is unclear, but it is believed that some of the minerals help settle the stomach.

I take medications with food. What can I do during fasting?

Certain medications may cause side effects on an empty stomach: Aspirin can cause stomach upset or even ulcers. Iron supplements may cause nausea and vomiting. Metformin, often prescribed for diabetes, may cause nausea or diarrhea. Talk to your physician about whether or not these medications need to be continued during your fast. Also, you can try taking your medications with a small serving of leafy greens, which is low in calories and may not disrupt your fast.

Blood pressure can sometimes drop during fasting. If you take blood-pressure-lowering medications, you may find your blood pressure becomes too low, causing light-headedness. Consult with your physician about adjusting your medications.

If you take diabetes medication, it's particularly important to talk to your doctor before beginning a fasting regimen—see the next question.

What if I have diabetes?

Special care must be taken if you have type 1 or type 2 diabetes or are taking diabetic medications. (Certain diabetes medications, such as metformin, are used for other conditions, such as polycystic ovary syndrome.) Monitor your blood sugar closely and adjust your medications accordingly. Close monitoring by your physician is mandatory. If you cannot be followed closely, do not fast.

Fasting reduces blood sugar. If you continue taking the same dose of diabetes medications, especially insulin, during your fast, your blood sugar may become extremely low, resulting in hypoglycemia. This can be a life-threatening situation. You must take some sugar or juice to raise your blood sugar back to normal, even if it means you must stop your fast for that day. You *must* closely monitor your blood sugar during your fast. If you repeatedly have low blood sugar, it means that you are overmedicated, not that the fasting process is not working. In the Intensive Dietary Management Program, we reduce medications before starting a fast in anticipation of lower blood sugar. But because the blood sugar response to a fast is unpredictable, close monitoring by a physician is essential.

Can I exercise while fasting?

Many people assume it will be difficult to exercise while fasting, and sometimes those with physically demanding jobs worry about fasting while working.

Yes, exercise demands extra energy from the body. However, the process of using stored food energy during a fast remains the same. The body starts by burning glycogen, the sugar stored in the liver. Since there is extra demand for energy during exercise, glycogen runs out sooner than otherwise. But your body generally carries enough glycogen for twenty-four hours, so it can sustain a fair amount of exercise before running out.

However, endurance athletes, such as Ironman triathletes, marathoners, and ultra-marathoners, do occasionally "hit the wall." Glycogen stores run out, leaving their muscles essentially running on empty. Perhaps there is no more indelible image of hitting the wall than the 1982 Ironman Triathlon, when American competitor Julie Moss crawled to the finish line, unable to even stand.

But even when our glycogen runs out, we're still carrying vast amounts of energy in the form of fat, and during fasting, our body switches from burning sugar to burning fat. Following a very low carbohydrate diet, or ketogenic diet, trains your body tissues to burn fat.

Similarly, exercising in the fasted state trains your muscles to burn fat. Instead of relying on limited glycogen stores, you can use almost unlimited energy from your fat stores. Muscles adapt to use whatever energy source is available. (This is the problem encountered by endurance athletes who hit the wall: they haven't adapted to using fat rather than glycogen for energy.) When we deplete our glycogen through fasting, our muscles learn to become much more efficient at burning fat. The number of specialized fat-burning proteins is increased, and the breakdown of fat for energy is enhanced. After training in the fasted state, muscle fibers show increased available fat. All these are signs that the muscles are training to burn fat, not sugar.

Does performance suffer? Not really. In one study, a three-and-a-half-day fast did not affect any measurements of athletic performance, including strength, anaerobic capacity, and aerobic endurance.

However, during the period when you are adjusting to the change from burning sugar to burning fat, you may notice a decrease in your athletic performance. This lasts approximately two weeks. As you deplete the body of sugar, your muscles need time to adapt to using fat. Your energy, muscle strength, and overall exercise capacity will go down, but they will recover. This process is sometimes called keto-adaptation. Very low carb diets, ketogenic diets, and training in the fasted state may all have benefits in training your muscles to burn fat, but your muscles do need time to adapt.

You can store far more energy in the form of fat than in glycogen, and for endurance athletes, the increase in available energy when they start burning fat is a significant advantage. If you are running ultra marathons, being able to utilize your almost unlimited fat stores instead of highly limited glycogen stores means that you won't "hit the wall," giving you a chance to win that race.

Since your body is relying on your fat stores, there's no shortage of energy during fasting, and you can and should do all your usual activities. There is no reason why exercise should stop during fasting. In fact, many elite athletes and endurance athletes train in the fasted state. The combination of low insulin and high adrenaline levels created by fasting stimulates the breakdown of fat and burning of fat for energy.

The six-foot-two-inch Academy Award–nominated actor Hugh Jackman routinely needs to gain and lose weight for different film roles. When he needed to lose twenty pounds for the film *Les Miserables*, he followed a low-carbohydrate diet. When he needed to pack on muscle for his role as Wolverine in 2013, he used intermittent fasting.

Can you exercise while fasting? Absolutely. The benefits include:

1. You can train harder due to increased adrenaline.

2. You'll recover from a workout and build muscle faster due to increased growth hormone.

3. You'll burn more fat due to increased fatty acid oxidation.

Train harder, build muscle, burn fat. Perfect!

I usually go 3–5 days with water, coffee (I use heavy cream), and bone broth with sea salt. My body has totally changed since I started fasting. I run a marathon every year, and this year was just amazing! I could keep my energy up the entire race and improved my time more than 30 minutes from last year. It was also my fastest time, even though I am 8 years older than when I ran my first marathon! Fasting definitely makes me healthier and much stronger!

—Kaori O., Houston, TX

Problems to Watch For

Close monitoring during fasting is essential for anyone with a health condition, but especially for diabetics. Blood sugar should be monitored at least four times daily if you are taking insulin. If you are feeling any symptoms of hypoglycemia, such as shaking or sweating, you should immediately check your blood sugar.

Blood pressure should be monitored regularly. This can be done at home with any of the widely available devices. Be sure to discuss routine blood work, including electrolyte measurement, with your physician. In addition to the usual electrolytes, we often monitor calcium, phosphorus, and magnesium levels.

Should you feel unwell for any reason, stop your fast immediately and see your doctor. In particular, persistent nausea, vomiting, dizziness, fatigue, high or low blood sugar, and lethargy are not normal with intermittent or continuous fasting and should raise a red flag.

Hunger and constipation, however, are normal symptoms and can be managed.

Feasts and Fasts: Understanding the Rhythms of Life

Celebrations with family and friends are integral to a life well lived. Every once in a while, we need to remind ourselves that life is sweet and we are lucky to be alive. And throughout human history, we've done that through feasting. The very act of eating is a celebration of life, and when we celebrate important events, we do so with a feast. Any diet that does not acknowledge this fact is doomed to failure. We eat cake on our birthday. We have feasts on holidays like Thanksgiving and Christmas. We prepare wedding banquets. We go to a nice restaurant on our anniversary.

We don't celebrate with birthday salad. We don't eat wedding meal replacement bars. We don't gorge on green shakes on Thanksgiving.

Like everything in life, weight gain is not constant; it's intermittent. Certain periods of life are associated with increased weight gain. This includes adolescence, when weight gain is part of normal development, and pregnancy, when weight gain is normal and necessary.

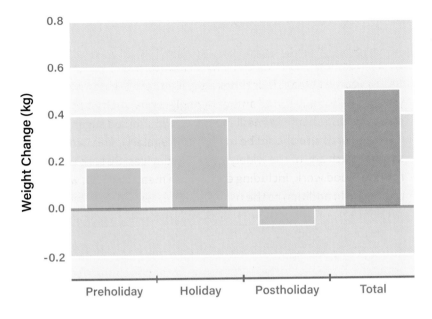

Figure 15.1. The majority of the year's weight gain happens during the end-of-year holiday period—as humans always have, we celebrate holidays with feasts.

Source: Yanovski et al., "A Prospective Study of Holiday Weight Gain."

Every year, the majority of the year's weight gain happens in a short period of time around the holidays. The period from Thanksgiving to New Year's covers only six weeks, but it accounts for roughly two-thirds of the year's 1.4-pound (on average) weight gain.

If weight gain is not uniform throughout the year, then weight loss efforts must also vary. You need a strategy that increases weight loss at certain times and maintains weight at other times. A constant calorie-reduced diet does not match the cycle of feast and fast and is thus doomed to failure.

There are times that you should eat a lot. There are other times that you should be eating almost nothing. That is the natural cycle of life. Most major religions acknowledge this by prescribing feasting at certain times—Christmas, for instance—and fasting at others—such as Lent. The ancient civilizations also knew this simple rhythm of life. When the harvest came in, they feasted. But they often fasted in the winter.

In Louisiana, food is a big part of our social fabric and heritage. Implementing fasting in my daily routine made me realize the importance of the "feast" from a totally different perspective. Without fasting, you simply don't truly understand the purpose of the celebration. Fasting has given me a deeper understanding of the feasts and celebrations we so enjoy here in our regional culture. And if we feasted with periods of fasting, like our Cajun ancestors, there would be a lot less obesity in our region.

—James B.,
Shreveport, LA

THE DAWN PHENOMENON

The occurrence of high blood sugar after a period of fasting is often puzzling to those not familiar with the Dawn Phenomenon. Why are blood sugars elevated if you haven't eaten for a while? This effect is even seen with prolonged fasting.

The Dawn Phenomenon, sometimes called the Dawn Effect, was first described approximately thirty years ago. It is estimated to occur in up to 75 percent of type 2 diabetics, although severity varies widely, and it's caused by circadian rhythms.

Just before awakening (around 4:00 a.m.), the body secretes higher levels of growth hormone, cortisol, glucagon, and adrenaline. Together, these are called the counterregulatory hormones—they counter the blood-sugar-lowering effects of insulin, meaning that they raise blood sugar.

These normal circadian hormonal surges prepare our bodies for the day ahead. After all, we are never quite so relaxed as when we're in a deep sleep. So these hormones gently get us ready to wake up. Glucagon tells the liver to start pushing out some glucose. Adrenaline gives our bodies some energy. Growth hormone is involved in cell repair and the synthesis of new protein. Cortisol, the stress hormone, increases as a general activator. All these hormones peak in the early morning hours and then fall to low levels during the day.

Since these hormones all tend to raise blood sugar as part of preparing for the upcoming day, we might expect that our blood sugar would go through the roof in the early morning. This does not normally happen. Why? Insulin also increases in the early morning to make sure that blood sugar does not go *too* high.

So even in nondiabetics, blood sugar is not stable throughout the twenty-four-hour circadian cycle. It's just that the early-morning rise in blood sugar is very small in nondiabetics, so it's easily missed.

But in people with insulin resistance, insulin has trouble putting the brakes on—the body isn't listening to its signals. Since the counterregulatory hormones are still working, blood sugar rises unopposed, resulting in higher-than-normal blood sugar early in the morning.

The same phenomenon is seen during fasting at any time of day. The hormonal changes during fasting include increases in growth hormone, adrenaline, glucagon, and cortisol—the same hormonal cocktail that's released before waking. As you fast, your insulin drops, but these hormones are still causing stored sugar to be released into the bloodstream, raising blood sugar levels.

Insulin moves the sugar from the blood, where it can be seen, into the tissues (liver) where it cannot be seen. It is like moving the garbage from your kitchen to beneath your bed. It smells the same, but you can't see it. When insulin levels drop, that garbage starts to move back to the kitchen, and we see higher blood sugar.

Is this rise in glucose in the morning or during extended fasting something worrisome? No, not really. Think of it this way: if you have fasted for two days and notice high blood sugar, where did that sugar come from? It could only have come from your own body, specifically the liver. That glucose molecule was always in your body, but you worry about it now because you can see it.

The Dawn Phenomenon, in which you see higher blood sugar during fasting, does not mean you are doing anything wrong. It's a normal occurrence. It just means that you have more work to do to clear out the stored sugar. And over time, fasting will do that.

What has happened in the past fifty years or so is that we have kept all the feasting but eliminated all the fasting. The normal balance has been perturbed, and obesity is the predictable outcome. If you feast, you must fast. That's really all there is to it.

But if obesity is the result of losing the fasting, what happens when you lose all the feasting? Well, life becomes a little less special. If you are the person at the wedding who won't drink, won't eat the cake, won't eat the full meal, won't eat the appetizers—there's a name for that: the party pooper. And nobody wants to be the party pooper.

Maybe you can keep it up for six months, or even twelve months. But forever? That's pretty hard to do. Life is full of ups and downs, and we need to celebrate the ups because the downs are right around the corner. But we must balance the periods of eating a lot with periods of eating very little. It's all a matter of balance.

Eating Out

Socializing over food plays a large role in our lives. We often get together with friends for a meal or coffee. This is normal, natural, and part of human culture worldwide. Trying to fight it is clearly not a winning strategy. Avoiding all social situations during fasting is not healthy and will likely lead to long-term noncompliance.

Fit fasting into your schedule, not the other way around. If you know you are going to eat a large dinner, then skip breakfast and lunch. One of the easiest ways to fit fasting into your life is to skip breakfast, since that's not a meal we socialize over as much as lunch or dinner. During workdays, skipping breakfast is easy to do without anybody noticing. This will quite easily allow you to fast for sixteen hours.

Missing lunch on workdays is also relatively easy: simply work through lunch. This allows you to slip in a twenty-four-hour fast without any special effort. There are also other added benefits. You are able to get more work done, so you might be able to leave earlier. Because you are staying busy, you may forget to be hungry. You also save some money. And unless you go out to lunch every day with the same crowd, nobody may even notice. Save money and time while getting thinner? Not a bad deal.

With 4 kids under 10, dinner at my house is always chaotic. By the time I've helped everyone with what they need (serving, cutting, more water, a dropped fork, etc.), I find myself eating as quickly as possible to finish by the time they are all done. When I'm fasting, I actually look forward to dinner. We have conversations about the day, things are relaxed, and I'm done when they are!

—Amberly C., Anderson, SC

References

A. M. Johnstone, P. Faber, E. R. Gibney, M. Elia, G. Horgan, B. E. Golden, and R. J. Stubbs, "Effect of an Acute Fast on Energy Compensation and Feeding Behaviour in Lean Men and Women," *International Journal of Obesity* 26, no. 12 (2002): 1623–8.

Christian Zauner, Bruno Schneeweiss, Alexander Kranz, Christian Madl, Klaus Ratheiser, Ludwig Kramer, Erich Roth, Barbara Schneider, and Kurt Lenz, "Resting Energy Expenditure in Short-Term Starvation Is Increased as a Result of an Increase in Serum Norepinephrine," *American Journal of Clinical Nutrition* 71, no. 6 (2000): 1511–15.

Delia E. Smith, Cora E. Lewis, Jennifer L. Caveny, Laura L. Perkins, Gregory L. Burke, and Diane E. Bild, "Longitudinal Changes in Adiposity Associated with Pregnancy: The CARDIA Study," *JAMA* 271, no. 22 (1994): 1747-51.

D. F. Williamson, J. Madans, E. Pamuk, K. M. Flegal, J. S. Kendrick, and M. K. Serdula, "A Prospective Study of Childbearing and 10-Year Weight Gain in US White Women 25 to 45 Years of Age," *International Journal of Obesity and Related Metabolic Disorders* 18, no. 8 (1994): 561–9.

Geremia B. Bolli, Pierpaolo De Feo, Salvatore De Cosmo, Gabriele Perriello, Mariarosa M. Ventura, Filippo Calcinaro, Claudio Lolli, et al., "Demonstration of a Dawn Phenomenon in Normal Human Volunteers," *Diabetes* 33, no. 12 (1984): 1150-3.

Jack A. Yanovski, Susan Z. Yanovski, Kara N. Sovik, Tuc T. Nguyen, Patrick M. O'Neil, and Nancy G. Sebring, "A Prospective Study of Holiday Weight Gain," *New England Journal of Medicine* 342 (2000): 861-7.

Joseph J. Knapik, Bruce H. Jones, Carol Meredith, and William J. Evans, "Influence of a 3.5 Day Fast on Physical Performance," *European Journal of Applied Physiology and Occupational Physiology* 56, no. 4 (1987): 428-32.

Karen Van Proeyen, Karolina Szlufcik, Henri Nielens, Monique Ramaekers, and Peter J. Hespel, "Beneficial Metabolic Adaptations Due to Endurance Exercise Training in the Fasted State," *Journal of Applied Physiology* 110, no. 1 (2011): 236–45.

K. De Bock, E. A. Richter, A. P. Russell, B. O. Eijnde, W. Derave, M. Ramaekers, E. Koninckx, et al., "Exercise in the Fasted State Facilitates Fibre Type-Specific Intramyocellular Lipid Breakdown and Stimulates Glycogen Resynthesis in Humans," *Journal of Physiology* 564 (Pt. 2) (2005): 649–60.

K. De Bock, W. Derave, B. O. Eijnde, M. K. Hesselink, E. Koninckx, A. J. Rose, P. Schrauwen, et al., "Effect of Training in the Fasted State on Metabolic Responses During Exercise with Carbohydrate Intake," *Journal of Applied Physiology* 104, no. 4 (2008): 1045–55, doi: 10.1152/japplphysiol.01195.2007.

Peter J. Campbell, Geremia B. Bolli, Philip E. Cryer, and John E. Gerich, "Pathogenesis of the Dawn Phenomenon in Patients with Insulin-Dependent Diabetes Mellitus—Accelerated Glucose Production and Impaired Glucose Utilization Due to Nocturnal Surges in Growth Hormone Secretion," *New England Journal of Medicine* 312, no. 23 (1985): 1473–9.

R. R. Wing, K. A. Matthews, L. H. Kuller, E. N. Meilahn, and P. L. Plantinga, "Weight Gain at the Time of Menopause," *Archives of Internal Medicine* 151, no. 1 (1991): 97–102.

Part Three
RESOURCES

FASTING FLUIDS

Only certain fluids can be consumed during fasting periods: water, tea and coffee (hot or iced), and homemade broth.

WATER

It is important to drink water frequently throughout the day when you fast. You can enjoy flat, mineral, or carbonated water.

What you can add to your water	What you can't add to your water
<ul><li>Limes</li><li>Lemons</li><li>Slices of other fruits (do not eat the fruit itself or consume fruit juice)</li><li>Vinegars (especially raw, unfiltered apple cider vinegar)</li><li>Himalayan salt</li><li>Chia and ground flaxseed (1 tablespoon in 1 cup of water)</li></ul>	<ul><li>Sweetened powders or drops (even if they're sugar-free)</li></ul>

COFFEE

You can consume up to six cups of coffee on a fasting day. The coffee may be caffeinated or decaffeinated. Black coffee is preferable, but you can add up to 1 tablespoon of certain fats to each cup of coffee if you wish (see the list of permitted fats below). Also, you can have unsweetened iced coffee: simply brew your coffee as usual and then refrigerate it or pour it over a cup of ice. For Bulletproof Coffee, see the recipe on page 264.

What you can add to your coffee	What you can't add to your coffee
<ul><li>Coconut oil</li><li>Medium-chain triglyceride oil (MCT oil)</li><li>Butter</li><li>Ghee</li><li>Heavy whipping cream (35% fat)</li><li>Half and half</li><li>Whole milk</li><li>Ground cinnamon, for flavor</li></ul>	<ul><li>Try to avoid low-fat and skim milks; whole milk is better</li><li>Powdered dairy products</li><li>Natural or artificial sweeteners of any kind</li></ul>

HERBAL TEA

You may consume unlimited herbal tea during your fasting period. There are a variety of teas that can help suppress your appetite, lower your blood sugar levels, or are otherwise beneficial.

Green Tea	• Good appetite suppressant
Cinnamon Chai Tea	• Can help lower blood sugar levels • Great for suppressing cravings for sweet foods
Peppermint Tea	• Good appetite suppressant • Good for alleviating GI discomfort, such as gas and bloating
Bitter Melon Tea	• Can help lower blood sugar levels
Black Tea	• Can help lower blood sugar levels
Oolong Tea	• Can help lower blood sugar levels

It's best to consume your tea black during your fasting periods, but you may add up to 1 tablespoon of certain fats to each cup of tea if you like (see the list of permitted fats below). You can also brew any herbal tea and refrigerate it or pour it over ice to make unsweetened iced tea. You can also make Bulletproof Tea by substituting tea for coffee in the recipe on page 264.

What you can add to your tea	What you can't add to your tea
• Coconut oil • Medium-chain triglyceride oil (MCT oil) • Butter • Ghee • Heavy whipping cream (35% fat) • Half and half • Whole milk • Ground cinnamon, for flavor • Lemon	• Try to avoid low-fat and skim milks; whole milk is better • Powdered dairy products • Natural or artificial sweeteners of any kind

HOMEMADE BROTH

It's not uncommon to experience some lightheadedness during your first few fasting periods. This is often caused by dehydration and decreased levels of electrolytes and can be easily remedied by consuming a good homemade broth. Both vegetable broth and broth made with the meat or bones from any animal or fish will work, but bone broth has one advantage: unlike vegetable broth, it contains gelatin, which is very beneficial for those who have arthritis or other joint problems. You may consume as much broth as you need to help you get through your fasting day. As time goes on, you will find that you need less and less broth during your fasting periods. See page 266 for a recipe for homemade bone broth.

What you can add to your broth	What you can't add to your broth
• Any vegetable that grows above the ground • Leafy greens • Carrots • Onions or shallots • Bitter melon • Animal meat • Animal bones • Fish meat • Fish bones • Himalayan salt • Any herbs (dry or fresh) and spices • Ground flaxseed (1 tablespoon per cup of broth)	• Vegetable puree of any kind • Potatoes, yams, beets, or turnips • Avoid store-bought broths, even organic

24-HOUR FASTING PROTOCOL

In this twenty-four-hour fasting protocol, you'll fast from lunch one day to lunch the next, or from dinner one day to dinner the next, three times a week. It also includes a daily sixteen-hour fast (which really just means skipping breakfast and eating only within an eight-hour window on nonfasting days; see page 203 for more). In the Intensive Dietary Management Program, we've found that this protocol works well for weight loss without urgency. However, if you prefer a less-intensive regimen, you could have just two twenty-four-hour fasts per week.

On eating days, we recommend you follow a diet that is low in refined carbohydrates and high in natural fats. Strive to eat only whole, unprocessed foods and avoid processed or prepared foods as much as possible.

In this protocol, you eat a meal every day, so it's ideal if you are taking medications that need to be taken with food. Also, it may be easier to fit into your schedule. For example, many people find that dinner is important not just as a time to eat but as a time to reconnect with spouses and children—on this schedule, you'll still have that family time. This sort of fasting schedule also fits easily into a typical work schedule.

In the example below, you'd fast from dinner on Sunday night until dinner on Monday night. If you finish dinner on Sunday at 7:30 p.m., then you would not have dinner on Monday until 7:30 p.m. The meals listed are suggestions for following a low-carb diet that's high in healthy fats.

	Sunday	Monday	Tuesday	Wednesday	Thursday	Friday	Saturday
Breakfast	FAST	FAST	FAST	FAST	FAST	FAST	FAST
Lunch	Strawberry and Kale Salad (page 292)	FAST	Arugula and Prosciutto Salad (page 288)	FAST	Tomato, Cucumber, and Avocado Salad (page 294)	FAST	Berry Parfait (page 262)
Dinner	Homemade Chicken Fingers (page 284); Avocado Fries (page 296)	Chicken Stuffed Bell Peppers (page 280)	Game Day Wings (page 282) with veggie slices and balsamic vinaigrette	Chicken "Breaded" in Pork Rinds (page 276)	Chicken Drumsticks Wrapped in Bacon (page 278) with roasted bell peppers	Steak Fajitas (page 286)	Grain-Free Cauliflower Pizza (page 274)

Sample of a three-times-per-week 24-hour fasting regimen. This shows fasting from dinner to dinner, but you could also fast from lunch to lunch.

36-HOUR FASTING PROTOCOL

In this thirty-six-hour fasting regimen, you'll fast for the entire day at least three days of the week. Unlike the twenty-four-hour fasting protocol, no meals are taken on fasting days, only fasting fluids (see page 254). Overall, this protocol is more effective for weight loss than the twenty-four-hour fasting protocol (page 257), and the longer fasting period is also better for reducing blood sugar and therefore may be better for those with prediabetes. Also, some people prefer the simplicity of fasting for the entire day, rather than eating one meal on fasting days, as on the twenty-four-hour protocol.

On eating days, we recommend you follow a diet that is low in refined carbohydrates and high in natural fats. Strive to eat only whole, unprocessed foods and avoid processed or prepared foods as much as possible.

In the example below, you'd fast from dinner on Sunday night until breakfast on Tuesday morning. If you finish dinner on Sunday at 7:30 p.m., then you would not eat again until breakfast on Tuesday morning at 7:30 a.m. You may consume breakfast, lunch, and dinner on nonfasting days.

	Sunday	Monday	Tuesday	Wednesday	Thursday	Friday	Saturday
Breakfast	Grain-Free Pancakes (page 268) with bacon	FAST	Simple Homemade Bacon (page 272); scrambled eggs	FAST	Mini Frittatas (page 270)	FAST	Berry Parfait (page 262); Bulletproof Coffee (page 264)
Lunch	Pear and Arugula Salad (page 290)	FAST	Tomato, Cucumber, and Avocado Salad (page 294)	FAST	Strawberry and Kale Salad (page 292)	FAST	Homemade Chicken Fingers (page 284); Avocado Fries (page 296)
Dinner	Grain-Free Cauliflower Pizza (page 274) with spinach salad	FAST	Chicken "Breaded" in Pork Rinds (page 276); Mustard Green Beans (page 298)	FAST	Steak Fajitas (page 286)	FAST	Chicken Stuffed Bell Peppers (page 280)

Sample of a three-times-per-week 36-hour fasting regimen. No meals or snacks of any kind are consumed on the fasting days, but you may consume any fasting fluid (see page 254).

42-HOUR FASTING PROTOCOL

In this forty-two-hour fasting regimen, you'll fast for the entire day at least three days of the week and skip breakfast every day, regardless of whether or not you are fasting. On fasting days, you are only allowed fasting fluids (page 254).

In the Intensive Dietary Management Program, we typically use this forty-two-hour fasting protocol for type 2 diabetes. The extended fasting period allows blood glucose and insulin more time to drop. However, if you are taking medications, you will need to consult your physician before fasting on this protocol, in order to avoid low blood sugar. While we want and expect blood sugars to drop, if you're overmedicated, they may drop too low, at which

point you may have no choice except to eat some sugar to raise it—which defeats the point of fasting.

On eating days, we recommend you follow a diet that is low in refined carbohydrates and high in natural fats. Strive to eat only whole, unprocessed foods and avoid processed or prepared foods as much as possible.

In the example below, you'd fast from dinner on Sunday night until lunch on Tuesday. If you finish dinner on Sunday at 7:30 p.m., then you would not resume eating until lunch on Tuesday afternoon at 1:30 p.m. On nonfasting days, you would consume lunch and dinner only, not breakfast.

	Sunday	Monday	Tuesday	Wednesday	Thursday	Friday	Saturday
Breakfast	FAST	FAST	FAST	FAST	FAST	FAST	FAST
Lunch	Arugula and Prosciutto Salad (page 288)	FAST	Chicken Drumsticks Wrapped in Bacon (page 278); carrot and celery sticks	FAST	Strawberry and Kale Salad (page 292); sliced avocado	FAST	Grain-Free Pancakes (page 268)
Dinner	Chicken "Breaded" in Pork Rinds (page 276); Roasted Cauliflower Rice (page 300)	FAST	Pear and Arugula Salad (page 290)	FAST	Steak Fajitas (page 286)	FAST	Chicken Stuffed Bell Peppers (page 280)

Sample of a three-times-per-week 42-hour fasting regimen. No meals or snacks of any kind are consumed on the fasting days, but you may consume any fasting fluid (see page 254). Breakfast is not consumed on nonfasting or fasting days.

7- TO 14-DAY FASTING PROTOCOL

This fasting protocol calls for fasting for seven to fourteen days consecutively. This means seven to fourteen days in a row without any meals or snacks. You are only allowed fasting fluids (page 254) during the fasting period.

In the Intensive Dietary Management Program, we typically use this protocol for severe diabetes or morbid obesity. In cases where control of diabetes and/or obesity is more urgent, we often suggest starting therapy with this protocol, then transitioning to a forty-two-hour fasting protocol (page 259). This protocol is also useful when hitting plateaus in weight loss and after periods of weight regain, such as the holidays and vacations (such as a cruise)—and knowing that you'll follow this protocol after a period of celebration can let you enjoy it without guilt.

This is a very intensive regimen and should only be attempted with the supervision of your physician. If you are taking medications, some of them will need to be adjusted prior to beginning the fast. (See page 242 for more information.) In this protocol, we also recommend the daily use of a general multivitamin in order to prevent micronutrient deficiency. Your physician may also want to monitor your bloodwork throughout the fast.

Remember, hunger does not progress. Day 2 is typically the hardest day on this regimen: studies of the hunger hormone ghrelin show that it peaks on day 2 of extended fasting and thereafter declines. Typically, each day gets easier. Most people remark after seven days that they feel they could have kept up the fasting forever!

Because of the risk of refeeding syndrome (see page 231), we do not often extend the fasting period past fourteen days. Instead, we recommend that you use an alternate-day fasting schedule such as the thirty-six-hour protocol (page 258) or forty-two-hour protocol (page 259) before repeating the seven- to fourteen-day fast. We recommend that you undertake seven-day fasts no more than once a month and fourteen-day fasts no more than every six weeks.

Remember that if at any point during the fast you do not feel well, for any reason, you should stop.

On this protocol, no meals or snacks are taken for at least seven full days—for example, starting on Sunday morning and continuing through Saturday night.

What?
RECIPES IN A BOOK ON FASTING?

YES.

Intermittent and extended fasting only form part of a healthy eating pattern. There are two parts to healthy eating: the part where you eat (feeding) and the part where you don't (fasting). We've covered fasting extensively, but a comprehensive plan requires both parts. Obviously, you cannot fast indefinitely, so eating a healthy diet is crucial. (See page 53 for more on a healthy diet.)

Megan Ramos is the program director of the Intensive Dietary Management Program in Toronto. She counsels hundreds of patients in both diets and fasting to achieve optimal health. Under her expert guidance, patients have reversed their obesity, type 2 diabetes, and metabolic syndrome. In many cases, patients have reduced or even eliminated their need for medications and learned how to maintain a healthy eating pattern for the rest of their lives.

In this section, Megan shares some of her favorite recipes, which can be incorporated into a fasting protocol like those on pages 257 to 259.

BERRY PARFAIT

PREP TIME: 15 minutes, plus 30 minutes to chill (optional) **COOK TIME:** — **YIELD:** 2 servings

INGREDIENTS

- ½ cup heavy whipping cream (at least 35% fat)
- 1 tablespoon 100% pure cocoa powder (optional)
- 1 teaspoon pure vanilla extract (optional)
- 6 almonds, crushed
- 6 walnuts, crushed
- 3 strawberries, diced
- ⅓ cup raspberries
- ⅓ cup blackberries
- 10 blueberries
- ½ tablespoon ground flaxseed (optional)
- ½ tablespoon chia seeds (optional)
- 1 teaspoon ground cinnamon, for serving (optional)

DIRECTIONS

1. Place the heavy whipping cream in a bowl and stir in the cocoa powder and vanilla extract (if using).

2. Using a hand mixer on medium, whip the cream until stiff peaks form, about 2 to 3 minutes.

3. *Optional:* For a nice chill on a hot day, place the bowl of whipped cream in the freezer for 30 minutes.

4. Stir the nuts and berries into the whipped cream.

5. Mix in the ground flaxseed and chia seeds (if using) and sprinkle the cinnamon over the top, if desired.

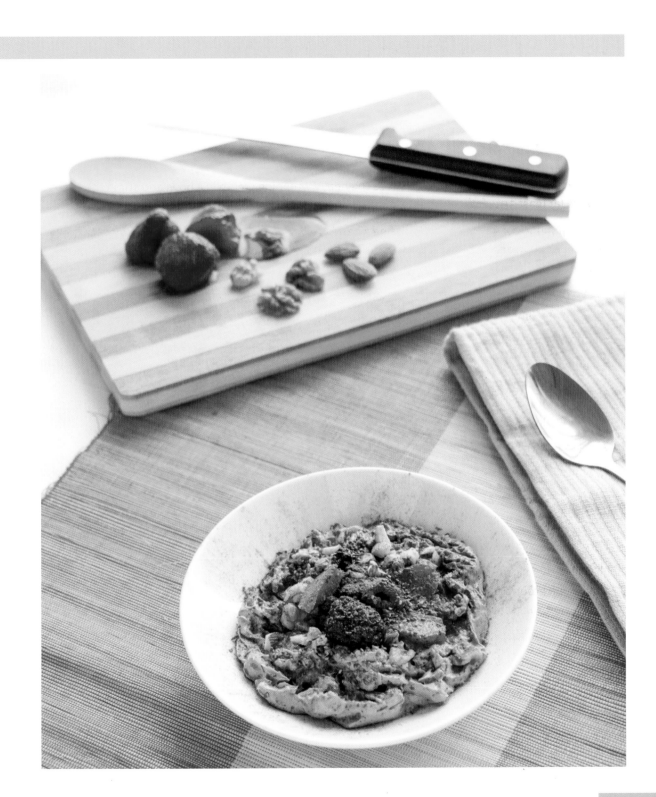

BULLETPROOF COFFEE

Bulletproof coffee has become very trendy in recent years. This can be consumed once a day on fast days to help you feel satiated. It's most helpful when consumed between the time you wake up and your regular lunch hour (if you are not eating lunch).

PREP TIME 2 minutes   **COOK TIME** —   **YIELD** 1 cup

INGREDIENTS

1 cup brewed coffee

1–2 tablespoons coconut oil or MCT oil

1–2 tablespoons butter

1–2 tablespoons heavy whipping cream (at least 35% fat)

DIRECTIONS

1. Add equal parts coconut oil, butter, and cream to the coffee.

2. Blend with an immersion blender until creamy.

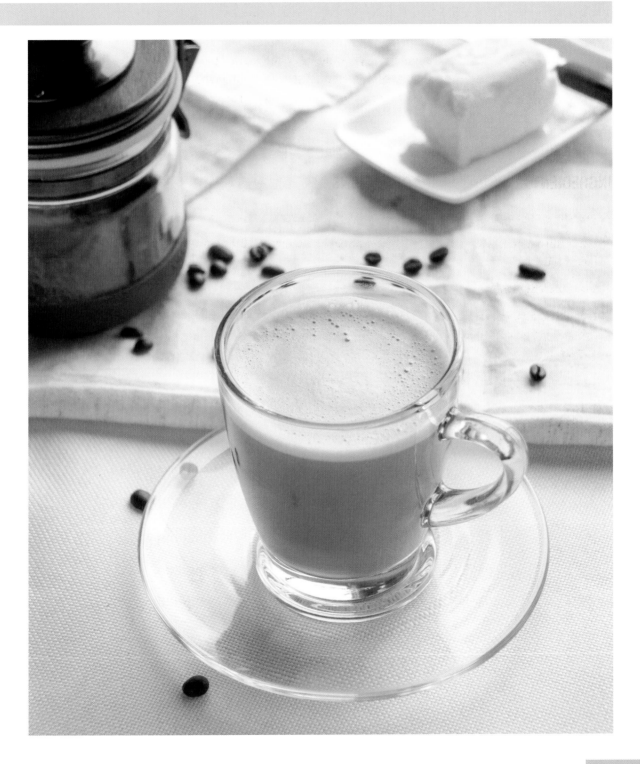

ESSENTIAL BONE BROTH

PREP TIME 10 minutes

COOK TIME 4 to 48 hours, depending on the kind of bones

YIELD 6 quarts

INGREDIENTS

6 quarts water

2 tablespoons raw, unfiltered apple cider vinegar

2 pounds animal bones (chicken, turkey, beef, pork, fish, or other)

1 medium onion, coarsely chopped

3 large carrots, coarsely chopped

10 stalks celery, coarsely chopped

1 red bell pepper, coarsely chopped

1 green bell pepper, coarsely chopped

1 tablespoon Himalayan salt

1 tablespoon black peppercorns

Fresh or dried herbs or spices of your choice (optional)

DIRECTIONS

1. Fill a stockpot with 6 quarts of cold water.

2. Add the vinegar to the cold water.

3. Place the bones into the water-vinegar mixture and let sit for 30 minutes. Prep your vegetables while the bones are soaking.

4. Add the onion, carrots, celery, bell peppers, salt, peppercorns, and any other dried herbs or spices (if using).

5. Place over medium-high heat and heat the water until it nearly boils, then reduce the heat to low. Let the broth simmer for 4 to 8 hours for fish bones; 18 to 24 hours for poultry bones; or 24 to 48 hours for beef or pork bones.

6. When there are 30 minutes remaining to cook, add any fresh herbs (if using).

7. Remove from the heat and let cool for 30 minutes. Then strain out the vegetables, bones, and fat.

8. Store in the refrigerator for up to 5 days or transfer to containers, ice cube trays, or muffin tins and store in the freezer for 3 to 4 months.

TIP

For more flavor, roast the bones on a baking sheet in a 300°F oven for 30 minutes before making the broth.

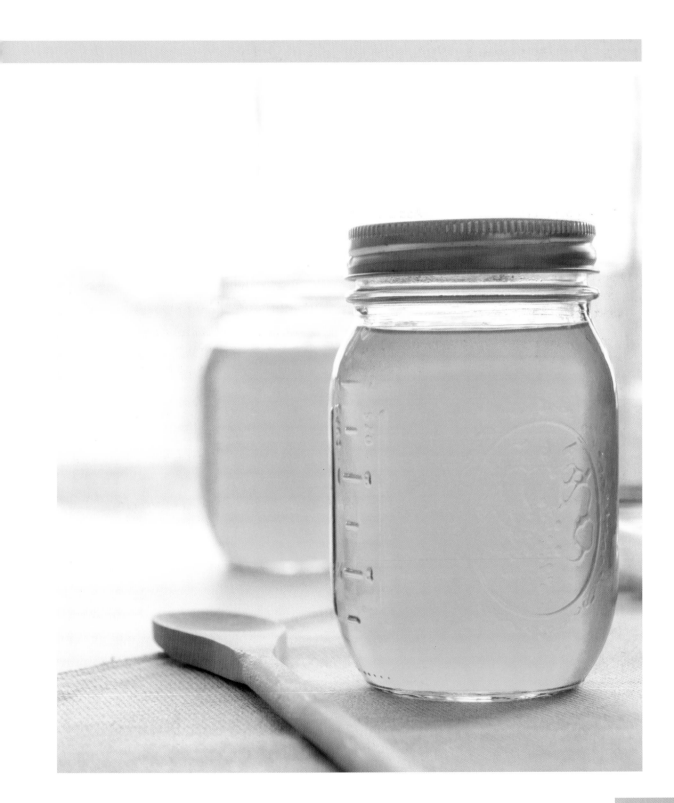

GRAIN-FREE PANCAKES

PREP TIME 10 minutes   **COOK TIME** 30 minutes   **YIELD** 4 to 6 pancakes (about 2 servings)

INGREDIENTS

2 eggs

½ cup heavy whipping cream (at least 35% fat), plus more for topping (optional)

1 teaspoon pure vanilla extract

½ tablespoon organic honey or erythritol

¼ cup coconut flour

½ teaspoon baking soda

¼ teaspoon Himalayan salt

1 tablespoon butter or coconut oil, plus more for topping (optional)

Ground cinnamon, for topping (optional)

DIRECTIONS

1. Preheat a skillet or griddle over medium heat.

2. In a small bowl, combine the eggs, cream, vanilla, and honey.

3. In a separate medium-sized bowl, combine the coconut flour, baking soda, and salt.

4. Slowly stir the wet ingredients into the dry ingredients.

5. Melt the butter in the skillet.

6. Pour in 2 or 3 tablespoons of batter to form pancakes about 3 inches in diameter. Cook for 2 to 3 minutes on each side, until golden brown. Repeat with the remaining batter.

7. Top the pancakes with whipped cream, butter, and/or cinnamon, if desired.

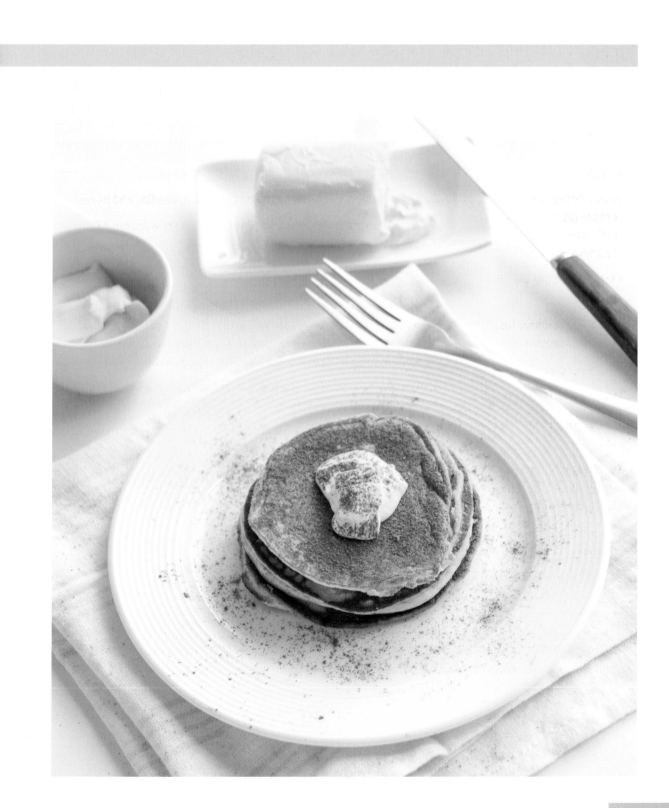

MINI FRITTATAS

PREP TIME: 15 minutes   **COOK TIME:** 20 minutes   **YIELD:** 6 frittatas
(2 to 3 servings)

INGREDIENTS

6 eggs

1 cup chopped spinach

12 cherry tomatoes, halved

⅓ cup diced red bell pepper

⅓ cup diced green bell pepper

½ cup green onions, finely chopped

½ cup grated cheddar cheese (about 2 ounces), plus more for topping (optional)

1 tablespoon Himalayan salt

1 teaspoon freshly ground black pepper

6 slices bacon

DIRECTIONS

1. Preheat the oven to 300°F. Grease a 6-cup muffin tin with butter or coconut oil.

2. In a medium-sized bowl, mix together the eggs, spinach, tomatoes, bell peppers, green onions, cheese, salt, and pepper.

3. Wrap a slice of bacon around the inside of each muffin cup. If there's any extra, trim it and add it to the egg mixture.

4. Fill each muffin cup about three-quarters full with the egg mixture. Top with cheese (if using).

5. Place in the oven and bake for 20 minutes, or until the tops are golden.

6. Remove from the oven and let cool for 10 minutes before serving.

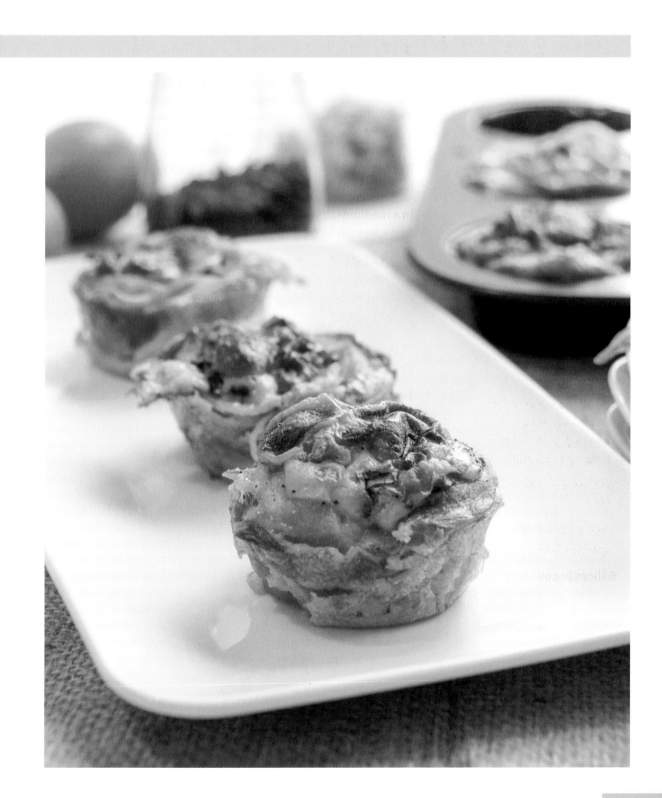

SIMPLE HOMEMADE BACON

PREP TIME: 15 minutes, plus 5 to 7 days to cure and 12 hours to chill   **COOK TIME:** 1½ to 2 hours   **YIELD:** 2 pounds of bacon

INGREDIENTS

2 pounds pork belly

⅔ cup Himalayan salt

2 tablespoons freshly ground black pepper

Dried herbs and spices of your choice (optional)

DIRECTIONS

1. Remove the skin from the pork belly with a very sharp knife. Try to keep the skin intact, in one piece, as you remove it.

2. Rinse the pork belly and pat dry with paper towel.

3. In a small bowl, mix together the salt, pepper, and any dried herbs and spices. Rub the mixture on both sides of the pork belly.

4. Place the pork belly inside a container with an airtight seal and store in the refrigerator for 5 to 7 days. The flavor becomes stronger the longer you cure it. Flip the pork belly over every day. (Make sure you wash your hands thoroughly before touching the pork belly.)

5. After 5 to 7 days, remove the pork belly from the refrigerator and rinse off the salt, pepper, and any other herbs and spices. Pat dry.

6. Preheat the oven to 200°F (90°C).

7. Place a roasting rack in a roasting pan. Place the pork belly fat side up on the rack.

8. Bake until the meat reaches an internal temperature of 150°F. This usually takes about an hour and a half to two hours.

9. Remove the pork belly from the oven and let it cool for 30 minutes.

10. Wrap the meat in parchment paper and store in the refrigerator overnight or for 12 hours.

11. Slice the meat to the desired thickness with a sharp knife. You can now cook your homemade bacon, or store it in the refrigerator for up to 5 days or the freezer for up to 2 months.

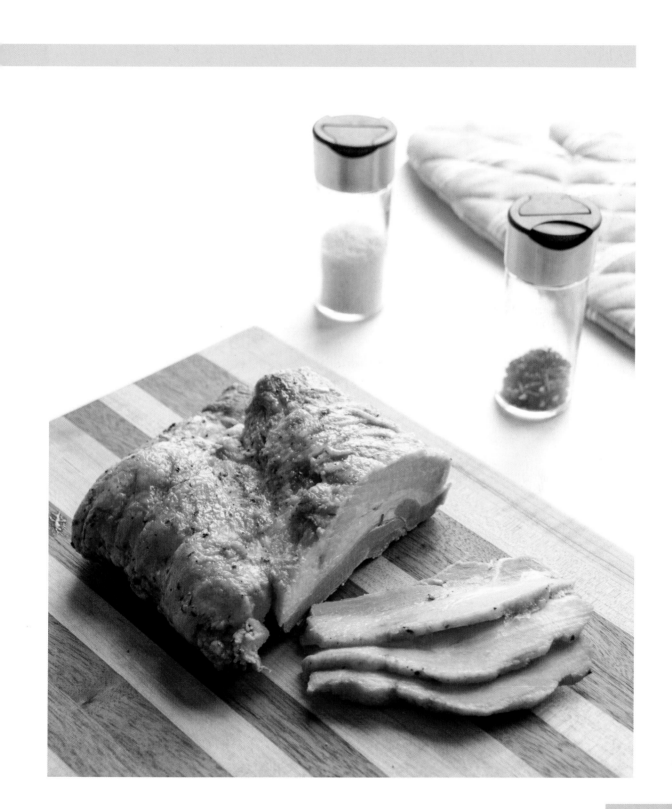

GRAIN-FREE CAULIFLOWER PIZZA

PREP TIME 10 minutes   **COOK TIME** 30 to 35 minutes   **YIELD** One 8-inch pizza (about 3 servings)

INGREDIENTS

- 1½ cups cauliflower florets (about 1 pound)
- 2 eggs, lightly beaten
- 1 teaspoon Himalayan salt
- 1 teaspoon dried oregano
- 1 teaspoon garlic powder
- Pizza toppings of your choice

DIRECTIONS

1. Preheat the oven to 400°F. Line a baking sheet with parchment paper.
2. Pulse the cauliflower florets in a food processor until finely chopped. Transfer to a large bowl.
3. Add the eggs, salt, oregano, and garlic powder and mix well.
4. Transfer the cauliflower mixture to the center of the prepared baking sheet and use your hands to form it into a pizza crust.
5. Bake for 20 minutes, or until lightly golden.
6. Add your desired toppings and bake for another 10 to 15 minutes.

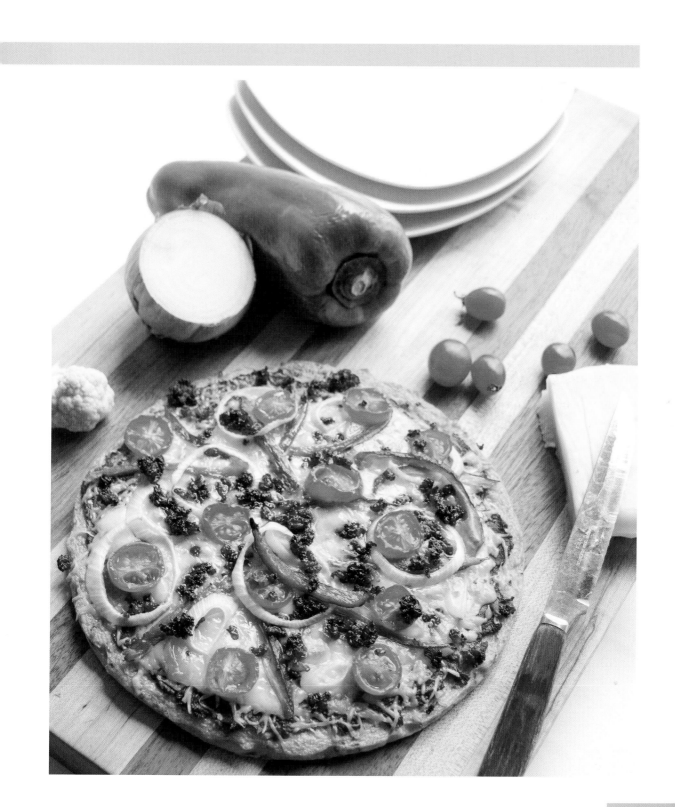

CHICKEN "BREADED" IN PORK RINDS

PREP TIME: 15 minutes   **COOK TIME:** 45 minutes   **YIELD:** 2 servings

INGREDIENTS

1¼ cup pork rinds

1 tablespoon Himalayan salt

2 teaspoons freshly ground black pepper

2 teaspoons smoked paprika

2 eggs

4 chicken thighs, skin on

DIRECTIONS

1. Preheat the oven to 375°F. Line a baking sheet with aluminum foil.

2. Place the pork rinds in a sealable plastic bag and crush them with your hands until they resemble bread crumbs. Add the salt, pepper, and smoked paprika to the pork rinds and shake until the spices and pork rinds are thoroughly mixed.

3. Whisk the eggs in a small bowl.

4. Place one of the chicken thighs in the egg mixture and leave it in for 10 seconds.

5. Transfer the egg-coated chicken thigh to the bag with the crushed pork rinds and seasonings. Shake until the thigh is coated, then remove and place on the prepared baking sheet.

6. Repeat with the rest of the chicken thighs.

7. Place the baking sheet in the oven and bake for 45 minutes, or until the chicken is golden brown.

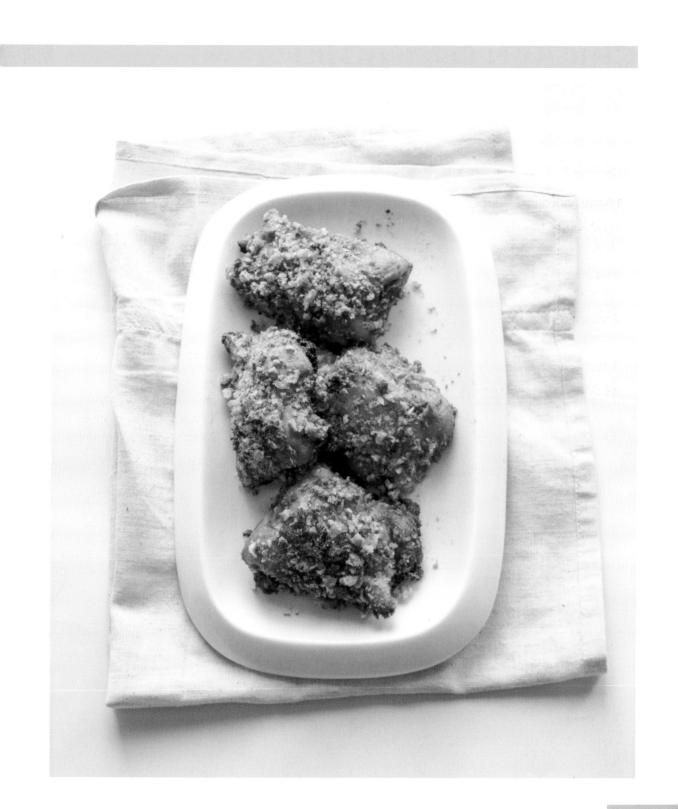

CHICKEN DRUMSTICKS WRAPPED IN BACON

PREP TIME: 5 minutes   **COOK TIME:** 45 minutes   **YIELD:** 2 servings

INGREDIENTS

4 slices bacon

4 chicken drumsticks

1½ teaspoons Himalayan salt

1 teaspoon freshly ground black pepper

DIRECTIONS

1. Preheat the oven to 400°F. Line a baking sheet with aluminum foil.

2. Wrap one slice of bacon around each drumstick, working your way from the bottom of the drumstick to the top. Place on the prepared baking sheet and season with the salt and pepper.

3. Bake for 45 minutes, or until the bacon looks nice and crispy.

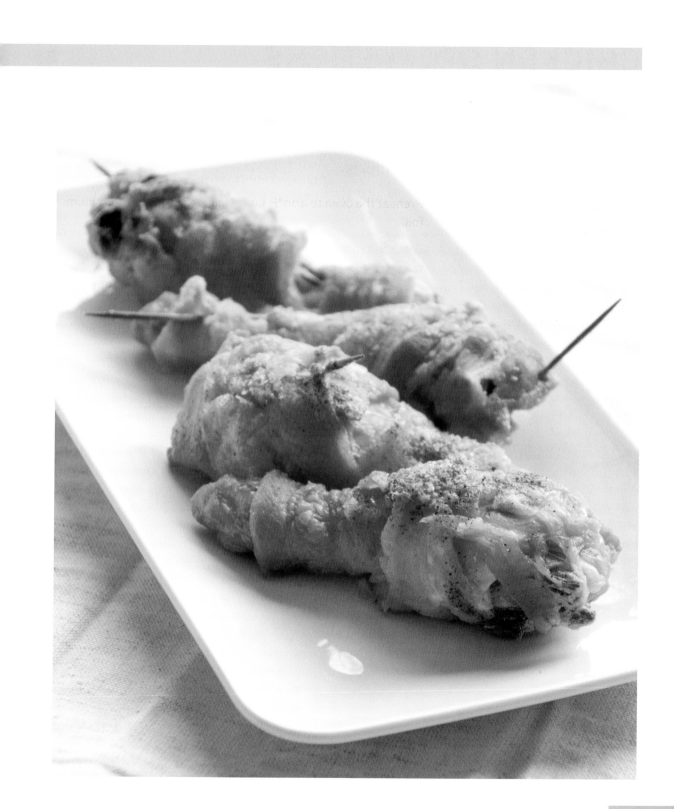

CHICKEN STUFFED BELL PEPPERS

PREP TIME: 10 minutes   **COOK TIME:** 1 hour 30 minutes   **YIELD:** 4 servings

INGREDIENTS

- 1 tablespoon butter
- 1 clove garlic, minced
- 1 small onion, diced
- 1 teaspoon Himalayan salt
- ½ teaspoon freshly ground black pepper
- 1 teaspoon smoked paprika
- 1 teaspoon chili powder
- 1 cup grape tomatoes, halved
- 1 pound ground chicken
- 3 eggs, beaten
- 4 large bell peppers, halved

DIRECTIONS

1. Preheat the oven to 350°F. Line a baking sheet with parchment paper.

2. Melt the butter in a skillet over medium heat. Add the garlic, onion, salt, pepper, smoked paprika, and chili powder. Sauté for 5 to 7 minutes.

3. Add the tomatoes and sauté for another 5 to 7 minutes.

4. Add the ground chicken and cook until golden brown, about 15 minutes, stirring occasionally.

5. Transfer the cooked meat mixture to a medium-sized bowl and slowly mix in the eggs.

6. Lay each bell pepper half cut side up on the prepared baking sheet. Pour the meat and egg mixture into the bell peppers.

7. Place the stuffed peppers in the oven and bake for 1 hour, until the peppers soften slightly.

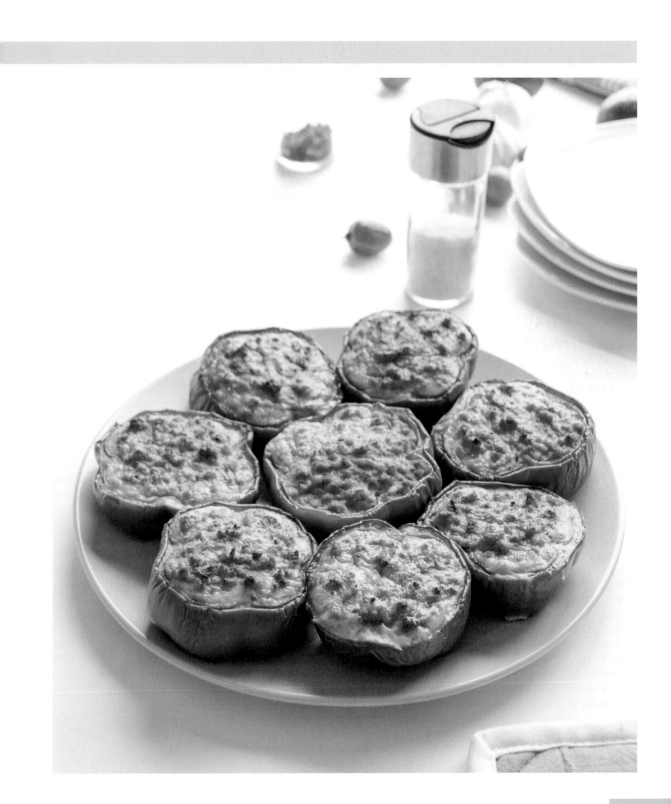

GAME DAY WINGS

PREP TIME: 5 minutes   **COOK TIME:** About 20 minutes   **YIELD:** 2 pounds of wings

INGREDIENTS

2 pounds chicken wings

1 tablespoon Himalayan salt

1 teaspoon freshly ground black pepper

1 tablespoon baking powder

1 teaspoon smoked paprika

1 teaspoon garlic salt (optional)

2 tablespoons coconut oil

2 tablespoons hot sauce (optional)

DIRECTIONS

1. Wash the chicken wings and pat dry.

2. In a small bowl, combine the salt, pepper, baking powder, smoked paprika, and garlic salt (if using).

3. Place the wings in a sealable plastic bag and add the spice mixture. Seal and shake the bag to coat the wings.

4. Preheat a skillet over medium heat. Melt the coconut oil in the warm pan.

5. Place the wings in the skillet and cover. Cook for 10 to 12 minutes.

6. Flip the wings and cook for another 10 to 12 minutes, until golden brown.

7. Remove the wings from the heat and let cool for 5 minutes.

8. Coat the wings with hot sauce, if desired.

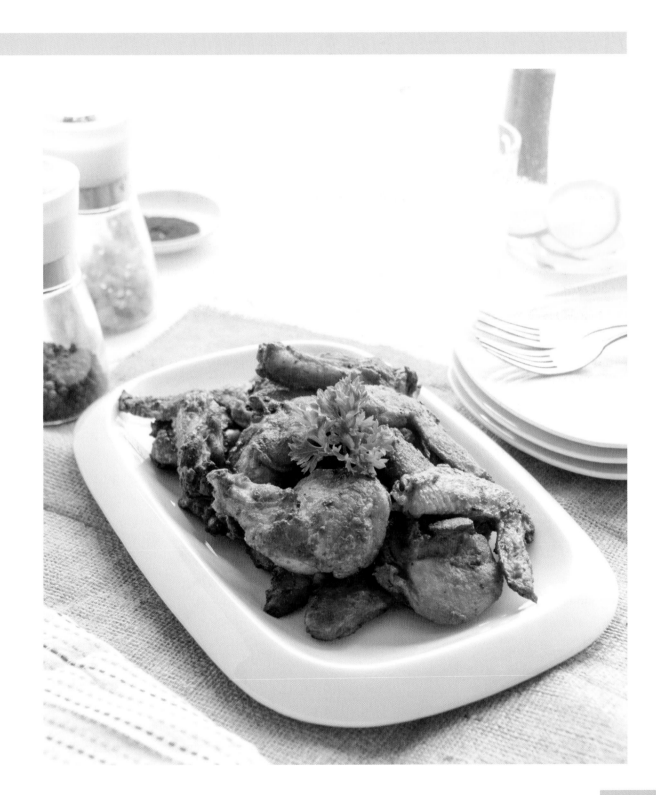

HOMEMADE CHICKEN FINGERS

PREP TIME 10 minutes   **COOK TIME** 20 to 30 minutes   **YIELD** 2 servings

INGREDIENTS

1 pound boneless chicken breasts, trimmed to 1 inch wide by 3 inches long

2 eggs

1 cup crushed pork rinds/ cracklings

1 tablespoon Himalayan salt

1 teaspoon freshly ground black pepper

1 teaspoon smoked paprika

1 teaspoon garlic salt (optional)

Hot sauce, for serving (optional)

DIRECTIONS

1. Preheat the oven to 300°F. Line a baking sheet with aluminum foil.

2. Wash the chicken fingers and pat dry.

3. In a small bowl, combine the crushed pork rinds, salt, pepper, smoked paprika, and garlic salt (if using). Pour the mixture into a sealable plastic bag.

4. In a medium-sized bowl, beat the eggs. Dip each chicken finger into the eggs to coat.

5. Add the egg-coated chicken fingers to the bag with the spice mixture. Seal and shake the bag to coat the chicken.

6. Place the chicken fingers on the prepared baking sheet and place in the oven. Bake for 10 to 15 minutes.

7. Flip the chicken over and cook for another 10 to 15 minutes, until golden brown.

8. Remove the chicken from the oven and let cool for 5 minutes before serving.

9. Serve with hot sauce, if desired.

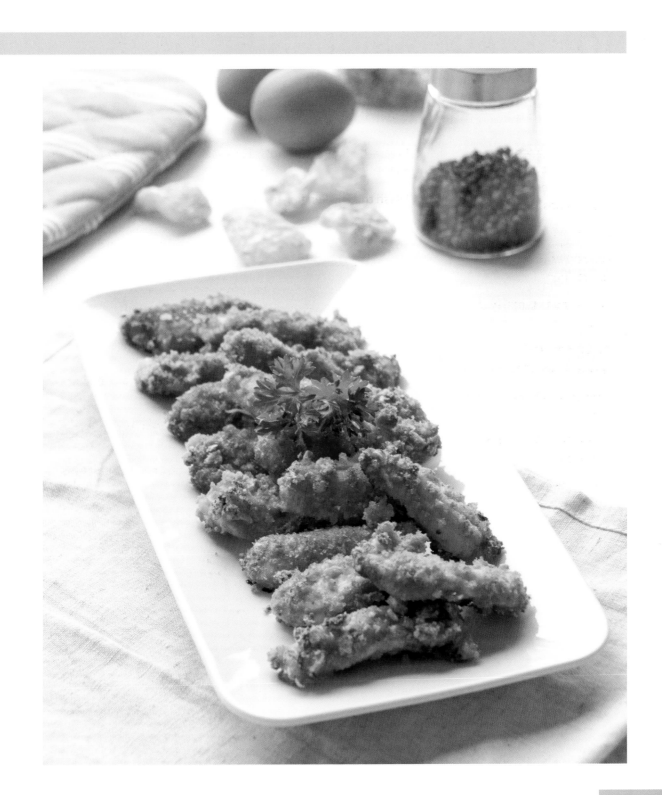

STEAK FAJITAS

PREP TIME 10 minutes   **COOK TIME** 20 minutes   **YIELD** 2 to 4 servings

INGREDIENTS

2 tablespoons butter, divided

1 red bell pepper, thinly sliced

1 green bell pepper, thinly sliced

1 yellow bell pepper, thinly sliced

½ onion, chopped

1 tablespoon Himalayan salt

½ teaspoon freshly ground black pepper

1 pound skirt steak

Large leaves of Boston lettuce (or other lettuce), for serving

FOR TOPPING (OPTIONAL)
Sour cream

Guacamole

Pico de gallo

Lime wedges

Grated cheddar cheese

DIRECTIONS

1. Heat a large skillet over medium heat. Melt 1 tablespoon of the butter in the skillet.

2. Add the bell peppers and onion and season with half of the salt and pepper. Cook, stirring occasionally, for 15 to 20 minutes, until the peppers are soft.

3. When there are about 10 minutes remaining for the vegetables, heat a second large skillet over medium heat. Melt the remaining tablespoon of butter in the skillet.

4. When there are about 5 minutes remaining for the vegetables, season the steak with the remaining salt and pepper and place it in the skillet with the butter. Cook for 3 to 5 minutes per side, until seared.

5. Remove both skillets from the heat.

6. Let the steak rest for 5 to 10 minutes before slicing. Cut into slices of the desired thickness.

7. Divide the sliced steak and vegetables into 2 to 4 equal portions and wrap each portion in a large lettuce leaf. Add your favorite fajita toppings and enjoy!

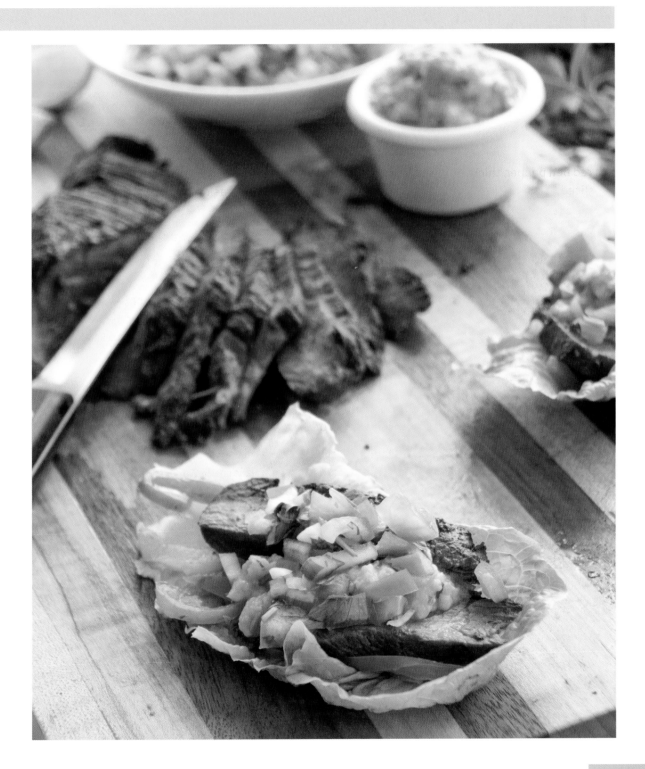

ARUGULA AND PROSCIUTTO SALAD

PREP TIME: 10 minutes   **COOK TIME:** —   **YIELD:** 1 serving

INGREDIENTS

2–3 cups arugula

6–9 thin slices prosciutto

½ cup chopped tomatoes

½ cup sliced olives

FOR THE DRESSING

1 tablespoon extra-virgin olive oil

1 teaspoon balsamic vinegar

DIRECTIONS

1. In a medium-sized bowl, toss together the arugula, prosciutto, tomatoes, and olives.

2. To make the dressing: Mix together the olive oil and vinegar.

3. Toss the salad with the dressing, or serve the dressing on the side.

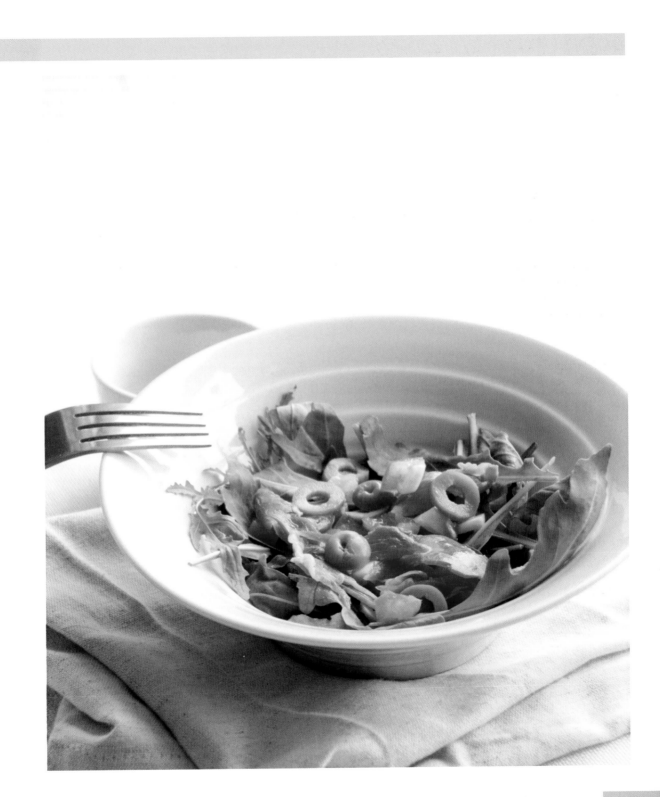

PEAR AND ARUGULA SALAD WITH PINE NUTS

PREP TIME: 10 minutes   **COOK TIME:** —   **YIELD:** 2 servings

INGREDIENTS

- 4 cups arugula
- 1 pear, thinly sliced
- ½ cup pine nuts
- ½ lemon
- ¼ cup extra-virgin olive oil
- Himalayan salt and ground black pepper

DIRECTIONS

1. In a large bowl, toss together the arugula, pear slices, and pine nuts.
2. Squeeze the juice from the lemon half over the salad.
3. Pour the olive oil onto the salad.
4. Season as desired with salt and pepper.

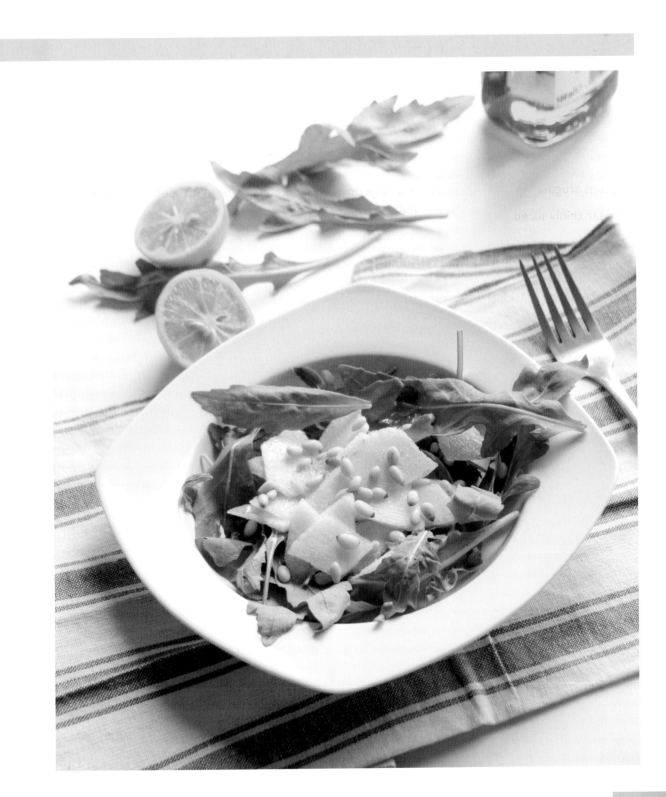

STRAWBERRY AND KALE SALAD

PREP TIME 10 minutes   **COOK TIME** —   **YIELD** 2 servings

INGREDIENTS

4 cups kale

12 strawberries, diced

1 cup walnuts

1 tablespoon balsamic vinegar

¼ cup extra-virgin olive oil

Himalayan salt and ground black pepper

DIRECTIONS

1. In a large bowl, toss together the kale, strawberries, and walnuts.

2. Pour the vinegar and olive oil over the salad.

3. Season as desired with salt and pepper.

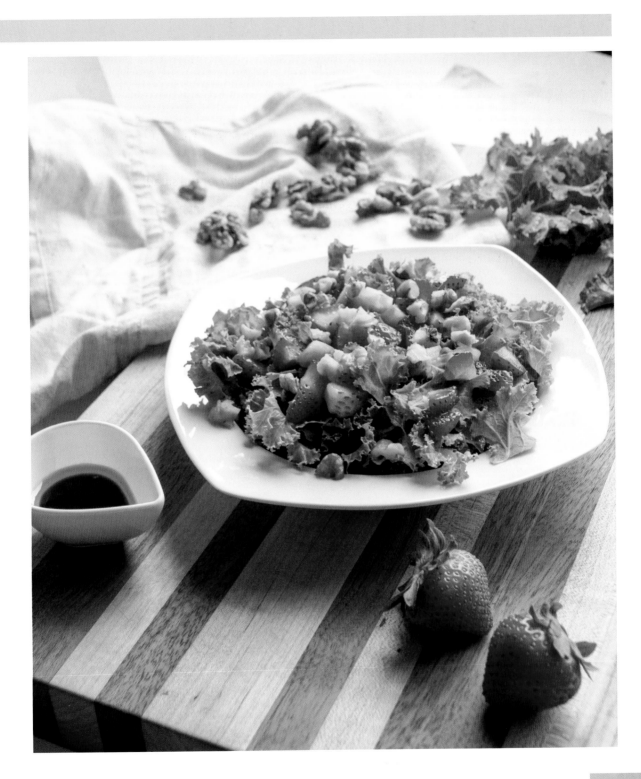

TOMATO, CUCUMBER, AND AVOCADO SALAD

PREP TIME 15 minutes   **COOK TIME** —   **YIELD** 2 servings

INGREDIENTS

- 2 cups diced cucumbers (about 1 medium cucumber)
- 1 cup halved cherry tomatoes
- 1½ cups cubed avocado (about 1 large avocado)
- 1 cup green olives, pitted and halved
- ½ cup feta cheese
- 1 tablespoon balsamic vinegar
- ¼ cup extra-virgin olive oil
- 1 teaspoon Himalayan salt
- ½ teaspoon freshly ground black pepper

DIRECTIONS

1. In a medium-sized bowl, toss together the cucumbers, tomatoes, avocado, and olives. Sprinkle the feta cheese on top.

2. Pour the vinegar and olive oil over the top and toss.

3. Season with the salt and pepper.

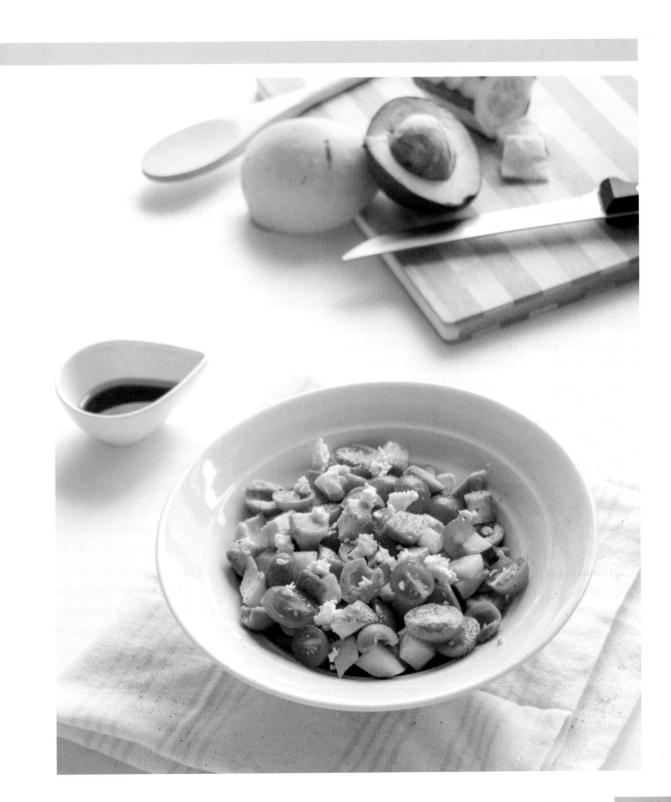

AVOCADO FRIES

PREP TIME 15 minutes   **COOK TIME** 15 minutes   **YIELD** 4 servings

INGREDIENTS

1 cup pork rinds

1 tablespoon Himalayan salt

Dried herbs and/or spices of your choice

Juice of ½ lime

1 egg

2 large avocados, cut into ¼-inch-thick slices

2 tablespoons melted coconut oil or butter

DIRECTIONS

1. Preheat the oven to 400°F.

2. Place the pork rinds in a sealable plastic bag and crush with your hands until they resemble bread crumbs. Mix in the salt and any dried spices or herbs.

3. Pour the lime juice into a small bowl. In a separate small bowl, whisk the egg.

4. Dip each avocado slice first in the lime juice, then in the egg. Let sit in the egg for about 10 seconds, then flip to coat the other side of the slice.

5. Place the egg-coated avocado slices in the bag with the crushed pork rinds and shake until the slices are covered in the pork rind mixture.

6. Pour the melted coconut oil into a baking dish and place the avocado slices in the dish.

7. Bake for 15 minutes, or until golden brown.

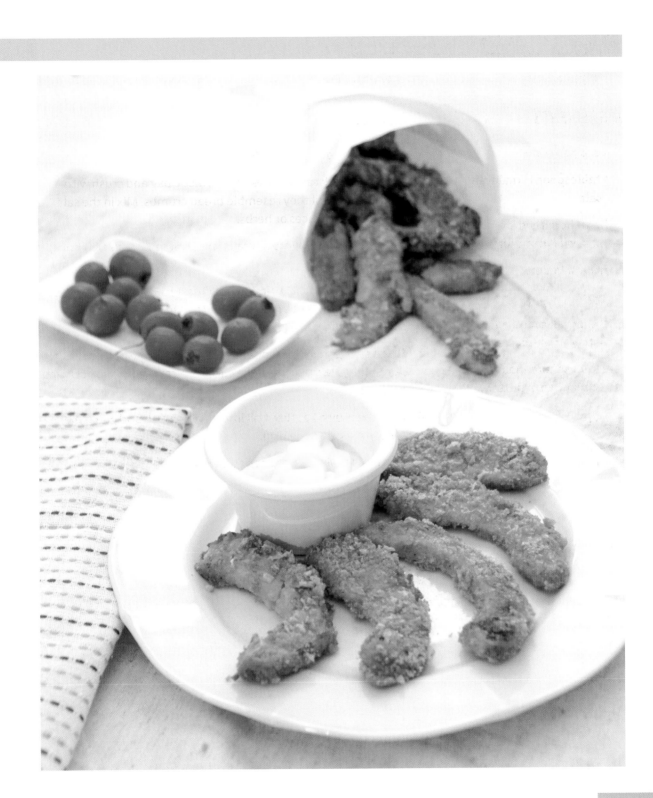

MUSTARD GREEN BEANS

PREP TIME: 10 minutes   **COOK TIME:** 10 minutes   **YIELD:** 4 servings

INGREDIENTS

- 1 pound green beans, trimmed
- 1 tablespoon extra-virgin olive oil
- 1 tablespoon mustard (any kind)
- Himalayan salt and ground black pepper

DIRECTIONS

1. Fill a medium-sized saucepan with enough water to cover the green beans and bring to a boil over medium-high heat. Add the beans and boil until crisp-tender, 3 to 4 minutes. Alternatively, you can steam the beans: fill a saucepan about three-quarters full with water and set a steamer basket on top. Bring the water to a boil over medium-high heat. Add the beans to the steamer basket and steam until crisp-tender, about 5 minutes. Remove from the heat.

2. Heat the olive oil in a nonstick skillet over medium heat for 5 minutes, then add the mustard.

3. Add the cooked beans to the oil and mustard mixture and cook for about 2 minutes, until well mixed and heated through.

4. Remove the beans from the skillet, season as desired with salt and pepper, and serve.

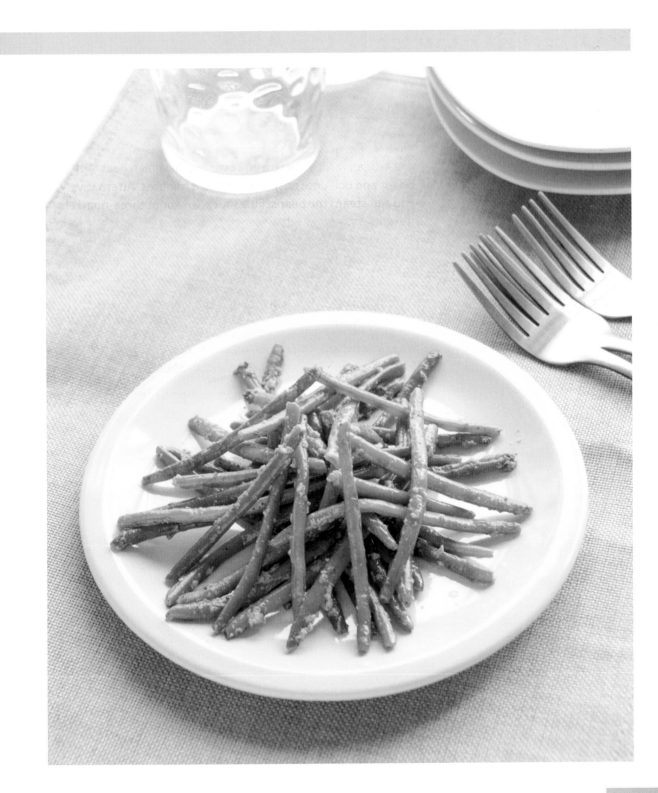

ROASTED CAULIFLOWER RICE

PREP TIME 10 minutes   **COOK TIME** 15 minutes   **YIELD** 2 servings

INGREDIENTS

1 head cauliflower

½ tablespoon Himalayan salt

Herbs or spices of your choice (optional)

DIRECTIONS

1. Preheat the oven to 200°F. Line a baking sheet with parchment paper.

2. Cut the cauliflower into florets and remove the stems.

3. Grate the cauliflower by hand or pulse it in a food processor until it looks like rice.

4. Spread the cauliflower rice on the prepared baking sheet and sprinkle with the salt.

5. Place the baking sheet in the oven and bake for 12 to 15 minutes, flipping every 5 minutes. Remove before the cauliflower rice starts to brown.

6. Add any desired herbs or spices.

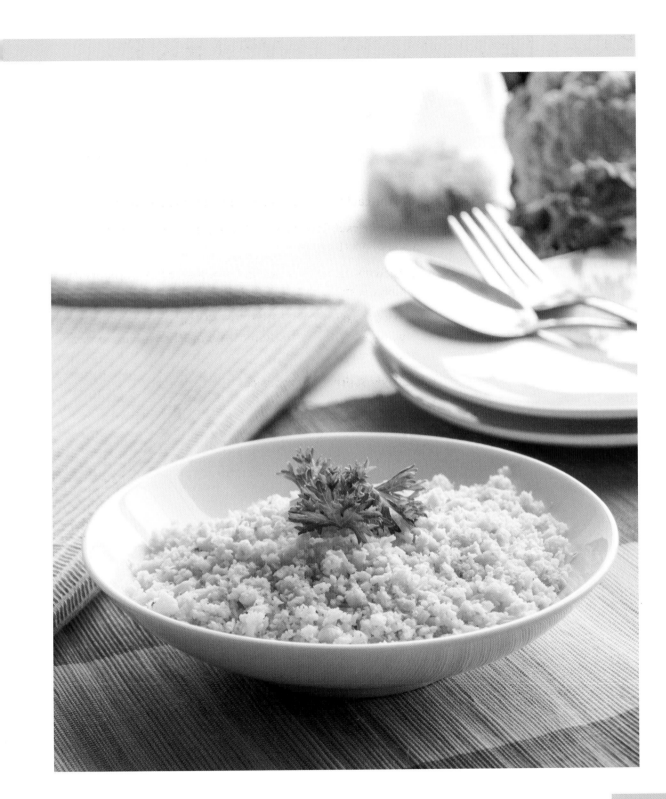

INDEX

A

adrenaline, 49, 51
aging, fasting and, 150–154, 181–182
Allen, Frederick Madison, 131–132
alternate-day fasting, 215
amyloid beta proteins, 153
ancient Greeks, 66–67
anorexia, 181
artificial fats, 56–57
Arugula and Prosciutto Salad recipe, 288
aspirin, 184
athletes, benefits for, 53
Avocado Fries recipe, 296

B

balance, 90–91, 246–247,250
Banting, Frederick, 132–133
bariatric surgery, 93, 119, 122–124
basal metabolic rate (BMR), 72–74
Benedict, Francis Gano, 225
Berger, Amy, 20, 69, 79, 140, 152, 170, 180, 194, 200
Berkhan, Martin, 53, 204
Berry Parfait recipe, 262
best practices, 196–198
bicarbonate, 228
The Biggest Loser (TV show), 101–106
bitter melon tea, 255
black tea, 255
Blaine, David, 233
"blaming the victim," 99
blood pressure, 246
blood sugar, 17, 78–80, 212, 226
Bloom, W. L., 68
BMI (body mass index), 180
BMR (basal metabolic rate), 72–74
BNDF (brain-derived neurotrophic factor), 149
body fat, 77, 107–111
body mass index (BMI), 180
bone broth, 198, 232, 256, 266
Bouchardat, Apollinaire, 130
bowel movements, 229
brain-derived neurotrophic factor (BDNF), 149
brainpower, fasting for, 147–150
breaking your fast, 237–238
breastfeeding, fasting and, 182–183
"bulletproof coffee," 194–195
Bulletproof Coffee recipe, 264

C

Cahill, Danny, 104
calcium, 49, 228
caloric-reduction approach, 100–101, 116–118
calories, 54, 107–109
"calories in, calories out" (CICO), 6–7
carbohydrates, 43, 54
cephalic phase, 172
chia seeds, as a natural appetite suppressant, 240
Chicken "Breaded" in Pork Rinds recipe, 276
Chicken Drumsticks Wrapped in Bacon recipe, 278
Chicken Stuffed Bell Peppers recipe, 280
children, fasting in, 181–182
chloride, 48–49, 50, 228
cholesterol
    about, 157–158
    high, 158–162
    lowering with fasting, 162–163
Cholesterol Clarity (Moore), 10, 25
CICO ("calories in, calories out"), 6–7
cinnamon, as a natural appetite suppressant, 239
cinnamon chai tea, 255
circadian rhythms, 204–208
coffee
    best practices, 197, 254
    Bulletproof Coffee recipe, 264
    as a natural appetite suppressant, 239–240
confusion, 242
constipation, 229, 240–241, 246
convenience, of fasting, 89–90
cortisol, 51, 124
cost, of fasting, 88
crankiness, 241
creatinine, 228

D

Dawn Phenomenon/Dawn Effect, 248–249
Denis, W., 225
diabetes. *See also* type 1 diabetes; type 2 diabetes
    about, 7–9
    early treatments for, 130–134
    extended fasting and, 229
    fasting with, 140–141, 185, 243

Dietary Guidelines for Americans, 54
diet(s)
    failure of, 86–87
    fasting and, 93
dizziness, as a common concern, 240
"dry fast," 195
dual-energy X-ray absorptiometry scan (DXA scan), 27
Duve, Christian de, 151
DXA scan (dual-energy X-ray absorptiometry scan), 27

E

Eades, Michael, 160
Eat, Stop, Eat (Pilon), 213
eating
    eating out, 250
    what happens when we eat, 43
The 8-Hour Diet (Berkhan), 204
electrolytes, 48–49, 228, 232
energy, 43
Epsom salts, 184
Essential Bone Broth recipe, 266
exercising, while fasting, 17, 243–245
exogenous growth hormone, 51
experiments, with fasting, 10–29
extended fasting
    about, 58, 225–227
    refeeding syndrome, 231–233
    7- to 14-day fasts, 230–231, 260
    two- to three-day fasts, 230
    what to expect during, 227–229

F

FAQs, on fasting, 241–245
fasted state, 44–45
fasting. *See also* extended fasting; longer-duration fasts; *specific topics*
    about, 39–41
    advantages of, 85–93
    aging and, 150–154, 181–182
    alternate-day, 215
    for brainpower, 147–150
    breaking your fast, 237–238
    combined with nutritional ketosis, 20–23
    cortisol and, 124
    diets and, 93
    disappearance of daily, 41–42
    effects of, 58
    experiments with, 10–29